I0422604

"THE REAL CURE FOR ARTHRITIS"

"THE REAL CURE FOR ARTHRITIS"

By Michael Burge

ISBN 978-0-557-20267-6

Table of Contents

1. Basic Understanding of Natural Healing 1

2. Why Our Traditional Diet Fails Us
    (Or Why The Body Breaks Down) 7

3. Other Remedies..13

4. Will Pride and Greed Overcome Truth? 19

5. What this Could Mean For Pro Athletes and Sports....................25

6. What This Could Mean For Everyone Else 29

7. The Cure: 1/2 Diet and 1/2 Habits 33

8. The Arthritis Foundation 1948 - 2009 and
    $400,000,000 - Where They Stand 39

9. I Need Grass Roots Funding Support 47

10. Relation Of This Cure To Other Diseases 51

11. My Vision for our Future..63

Disclaimer

I'm not a Dr., but am exercising my First Amendment Rights of Free Press & Speech. In light of the facts, no Significant Breakthroughs [Cures or Quantum Leaps] have been made in the 60 year and $400,000,000 tenure of the Arthritis Foundation, along with countless "Trillions of Dollars" spent by Americans during this time for medications, therapy, other research and development, work production lost, etc. ad-infinitum!! Most importantly though is the pain, suffering, hopelessness, & humiliation endured by our people [& all people of the world] etc.. which a dollar amount cannot be put upon!! I offer this Empirical Knowledge, gleaned from a Strong Faith and Persistent Research over the last 22 years, since my Paradigmatic Discovery in 1987!! But really their roots stem back into the Revolutionary 1960's, when I began 'Hearing the Beat of a Different Drum' and 'Took a Journey Down the Road Less Traveled' !! I've followed a Light that was always there, even as My Path had many Hills and Valleys!! Michael Burge 10/11/2009

The 3rd Millennium (of Peace) has already begun,

But we have missed the starting gun!

The status quo is not going to cut it,

Til you Follow your Hearts and the Holy Spirit!

Dedication

To my mom, Jean Burge, who had an unfulfilled dream to write a book! But her Prophecy in her Poem "The Better Yet Seeds" has finally come true!! Thanks for keeping in touch~

My dad, Ernest Burge, for always providing the financial stability, along with strict and challenging guidance in my life! Now our connection is surely Science Fiction~

To Grandma, who kept the house in order and whose own struggle with Arthritis created more hardship in her life than she deserved! And the great sense of humor of Paw Paw, who delighted my young life, & helped my own sense of humor!

To Teresa, my older sister, who left this Earth far too soon... thanks for watching over me then and now!! And let's see... oh yeah, my younger sister Donna... she like Dad was the Champion in the Family - excelling in school, sports, and finances... thanks for your Help & Inspiration!!

The toughest and most grueling part of this Solitary Quest, has been the Lack of Peers in the Understanding of how the Diet (and subsequent habits) and Nature and God all Interrelate with each other to Sustain Humanity in the greatest degree possible!! Were it not for my Guiding Spiritual Friends in the Dream World and of course God, all this probably would not have been possible!!!

And finally, Dedicated to the Reunion of God's (or buy whatever name one has learned or chooses to call the Good and Holy Creator of All) Family on this Earth, our Home, and once and for all the Beginnings of a True Peace!!!

CHAPTER 1

Basic Understanding of Natural Healing

In the King James' version of the Bible, Genesis Chapter I, verse 29 and 30: "And God said, *Behold I have given you every green herb bearing seed, which is upon the face of the earth, and every tree in which the fruit of the tree yielding seed; to you it shall be for meat. And to every beast of the earth, and every fowl of the air, and everything that creepeth upon the earth, wherein there is life, I have given every green herb for meat;* and it was so." The Bible is a Great Book that presents a widely accepted view of Creation & basically tells of earlier Tribes of Humanity, their relationship with each other and God; and especially many Rules of Truth that are accepted in any culture, faith or nation–'Love One Another' being amongst the highest! We read the words of the Bible or any Holy Book, and they teach and describe things for us; but as many (but not enough) know, beyond the words is actual Experience and Relationship with God and Each Other in Higher & Deeper Levels of Being!! When one experiences Unconditional Love or union and understanding with God, you would see how a commandment "Thou Shall Not Kill" pertains to all life, with a volition of its own! The Earth Animals, which are thought to be here for the purpose of Feeding the Humans, have a consciousness behind those eyes not unlike our own, just different, and many times, more evolved in ways, as they are naked to the world and its elements, and really can't indulge in the things that humans do that are detrimental to our well-being! The Bottom Line: cancer, heart attack, arthritis, diabetes, etc. ad-infinitum still plague humanity as they have for eons... God doesn't make Design Mistakes!!! I say that the Main Root of these Common Sicknesses lie in how we feed ourselves [w/ the animals & their by-products], along w/ our subsequent habits, thoughts, & feelings!!

"Common Sense" is an attribute of the mind and heart in which one inherently knows something to be true. Many will say to me after

I offer the commandment, "Thou shall not kill," as one reason for not eating meat, that you kill a vegetable or fruit when you eat it ..how absurd, don't be so foolish & stubborn! Your health, life enjoyment and Earth's Future depends on a mass recognition of new changes, which in turn will evolve into higher ways in all areas as we once again realize "We are All God's Family." Take the time to consider "We are All God's Family" ... it's truth beyond the illusion we are mostly caught up in. Look clearly at our current situations: sickness and disease is widespread with nothing hopeful in sight, but rhetoric stringing the hopeful out; even for the steadily working ones without major problems, there are many things that plague them from being well-rounded spiritually, mentally, physically, etc.; dissension between the generations and sexes is disappointing much less disenchanting; alcoholism, drug misuse, and crime all have some of their roots in diet (as I will relate to later); wars and rumors of war, earthquakes, famines and floods more and stronger than ever before – for those that have Eyes to See and Ears to Hear, don't be alarmed, for the end is not yet to come ... sound familiar??!! I say don't let it come, the Earth is our Home and We are All God's family!! Get out of the "Holy Illusion" that the "End Time" is about Death and Destruction except for the Saved (many Saved have perished before, but in the end it's All between each Individual & God); and let us clean up ourselves and our messes and help bring a Heavenly Glow back to the Earth Our Home and Each Other!!!

Use God as a Common Denominator for any problem or quest, and weigh it out with Truth which is Common to All our Hearts and Souls! Life is certainly an Adventure, a Challenge, & a Soul Education, but is not meant to be Impossibly Hard ... though as one of its basic rules states "We Reap what We Sow," and we have really Created a Predicament, haven't we??!! Just like when one becomes lost in the woods or the city, for that matter, reversing your steps or backtracking is usually the best way to solve the situation. Likewise, the basic premise in Natural Healing is undoing some of what has been done.

I believe a totally Raw Food Diet is the most superior diet one can have! A raw food diet is any food that comes out of the Earth – fruits, vegetables, nuts, melons, etc. and is eaten as is without cooking, steaming, etc. Of course you can use spices, seasonings, herbs, oil, and water to enhance the flavor and energy. The most important thing about a raw food diet is its Live Enzymes and Energy, going into a

Live Body, equals quick digestion and assimilation and better and more balanced energy... it's Powerful Food!! Now if one is on a traditional diet, or even a beginning vegetarian diet, a raw food diet, is still a good ways off! Better to make small and consistent steps, than big steps and backslide later. Here is an important part in Natural Healing–feed and clean the body right and it knows how to heal itself ... you eat your food–you don't have to tell it where to go and what to do; it already knows, God Designed it that way!! Diet alone, is not by any means a cure-all; you could have the best diet in the world, but if you have poor digestion or clogged up assimilation or elimination, you will still have problems. Likewise, if you are emotionally bound up or spiritually lost, you will never obtain optimum health and vitality!!

Some other forms of natural healing are: massage, rebirthing, prayer, fasting, meditation, listening to your dreams, chanting or singing, affirmations, consistent exercise, crying, relaxing, friendship and love. Natural Healing could be defined as correctly diagnosing your situation and helping your body to work out its problems; ideally without pharmaceuticals, surgeries, etc. (although sometimes these are necessary and we should be thankful for them, but they definitely need to coordinate with what I speak of in this book). Then, maintaining and evolving an ever-increasing healthy lifestyle... don't lag around too long in your 'comfort zones'!! Another important aspect of natural healing is reversing the steps that attributed to your condition. A general example of this could be upon awaking in the morning you first have one or two cups of coffee and then a traditional breakfast (if any) of any of the following: eggs, cheese, milk, bacon, sausage, refined pancakes or oatmeal, and more coffee. Then mid morning coke and/or donuts/ candy bar, and more coffee (and very little water or mental rest or relaxation). For lunch – burgers, pizza, or other gunky fast foods and cokes. Then, an afternoon coke and/or candy bar. Then, without any rest periods after work, hustle to your next concerns. Then perhaps a few beers, glasses of wine or liquor, again with little or no water. And for supper, the traditionally big meal of the day, another heavy gunky type meal mostly of meat, cheese, sticky flour products, cooked vegetables, and a very low percentage of raw, live enzyme food; then the desert! Obviously, the above is very general and covers a broad possibility of situations. I have heard of two pots of coffee being drunk a day, then more alcohol, and add in cigarettes, and arthritis will strike soon and hard!! To reverse the above situation and begin the cure, upon arising drink a good glass of water, add in some deep breathing, Remembering & Interpreting Dreams, a hot bath, spiritual reading & meditation {I know that Time is HUGE, but 5 minutes or so of each is 30 minutes} and Wake Up before getting so busy. Eat some fresh seasonal fruit with a whole grain cereal and try pouring orange juice over the cereal sometimes instead of cow's milk [or substituting a soy or nut milk], and adding some raisins instead of another teaspoon of white sugar. Go ahead with a cup of coffee, but a little less strong [or some black tea – ½ the strength of coffee], and maybe with ice during the warmer months. I am not much, anymore, for in-between meal snacks (usually they are more of the junk food variety anyway), probably more and smaller meals would be better for those that snack too much. However, in-between meals, it's very important to have two to three glasses of water spaced in, if you eat your meals four to six hours apart. Adequate water is very necessary for digestion, assimilation and elimination, not to mention helping to keep the body fluid! Coffee, alcohol, cigarettes, and too much tea, drastically depletes the body of this resource & dehydrates it!! Now for lunch, which should be the largest meal of the day, there are endless varieties of salads that can be made. Be sure to make them colorful, like the rainbow. A good balance to strive for is one-half raw food and one-half cooked food. In Chapter 2, I will make some recipe suggestions that are not too big a jump from traditional ways. If possible, after eating lunch, take a ten or fifteen minute walk or a short nap, depending on what your body is telling you or what you need to do. Again have a few glasses of water during the next couple of hours and you will also find this will pick you up, as it helps with digestion and assimilation, etc.; so, many times you won't need the extra coke, coffee or candy bar. However, if after say two hours or so you feel of a need for a "sweet charge", get an apple or a piece of cantaloupe or something in season and include a glass of water also. After work and other important concerns, if alcohol is your inclination to help unwind, take in less and have a glass of water along with and/or in-between drinks! And finally for supper, don't eat too late, try to eat one-half raw and one-half cooked (but less food than lunch), have plenty of water and after eating take a leisurely stroll. Allow two to three hours between supper and sleep. This is a good start and after you become accustomed to it, take it a little further to the vegetarian way; or if you are already a vegetarian a little closer to the vegan, then the raw food diet way. This is what I call reversing your steps in diet and routines.

One did not just begin drinking two pots of coffee first thing in the morning, having a coke and candy bar two hours after breakfast, smoking a pack of cigarettes daily, or drinking a six-pack of beer in the evening. The most secure way to better health is cutting back on the detrimental things and replacing them with healthier alternatives (concerning diet and routines)! Be moderate yet firm in your attempts while you are learning new habits and the ways they affect you. Find healthy people to advise you in ways that are new or different to you. Two points that I cannot emphasize enough – Pray for Guidance and Listen to your Dreams ... it is Your Life, use all your Available Gifts!!

CHAPTER 2

Why Our Traditional Diet Fails Us (Or Why The Body Breaks Down)

God doesn't make Design Mistakes. If you have had a Holy Experience with God, you can relate to being Humbled to your knees and tears, and thankfulness, & or a Transcendent Understanding ... if you haven't or have Doubt in a Belief, go off by yourself, settle down, and Give Prayer a Chance; God is always there!! For those who believe in God take your understanding a step further. An often asked question "Why did God let them suffer or die from such a slow, horrible death?" and then you give up, saying God has his reasons or the doctors and scientists with a little more money and time will find a cure, it's just around the corner. With all due respect for their intent and modern technology that's what I have been hearing since I was a child in the 1950's; it started with a cure for the common cold ... there isn't one, it's just the body throwing off much of the junk we feed it, after a fever comes from a plugged up and toxic body trying to clean itself. Yet we try to stop this process with medicines that further complicate our health, without letting the body complete it's natural process. God let's this happen so we learn, much of the time through our suffering, pain and ignorance, like a child learning how to walk. If the Doctors and Scientists really care, they must be open to Natural Healing!

"Seek and You Will Find," is one of the most inspiring challenges we could ever have! Life is not solely for the purpose of being "Saved," as some would perpetrate their insecurities on the whole; but to experience and learn from... Heaven can Wait, Live Your Life... Live it Well, & Heaven will be there @ the End!! Seeking is an attitude and a cooperation of all; we have got to find the answers for the common good! With so much competition, pride and greed it's definitely an up-hill battle. Also, many of the laws today and public opinion are stacked against natural healing, alternative they call it, they make it sound second-rate! Well Doctor, M.D., Phd., A through Z's, try a fast for a few days some time and see what your addictions really are; if you can do it great, see how you will feel and pass it on!

So, looking at the big picture, and starting from America's past, common talk has been how healthy our ancestors were; though many only lived 40 years!   Was this because of the lack of advanced technology, etc.? Maybe in part, but God's laws transcend time and space and violating its accords will never work! A gas engine cannot run well on one-half diesel and one-half gas. Humanity (and the animals) cannot prosper fully with a traditional diet that contains animal products, especially meat (the slaughtered animals)! This is the main reason why the widespread (throughout history as we know it) sickness and disease with no real cures in site! There have been some "plagues" we've overcome such as polio, typhoid, etc., with the cure attributed to a vaccine. Perhaps, we were way down in oppression, poor diet, too much work without hope ... I recall <u>many</u> pictures from American history that showed what a tremendous struggle it was! Not much of the Harmony that God Smiles at, though! It's in the history books; most probably have vague recollections, but haven't added it up! Eat a natural diet according to the seasons (no animal products or dairy -- why should a human suckle from a cow, her milk is meant for her calf, you don't cross species -- common sense); work hard and smart; rest several times a day; exercise; have friends and love; pray and meditate; have fun; share; and with satisfaction sleep and dream well.

So if it is True that animals were never "Ordained" by God to be food for humans or each other, and you have a traditional animal based diet, therein lies one of the major problems of your Health and Sanity!!! Obviously, if something were not meant for intake and one does so anyway, a malfunction at some point will begin to occur, i.e. common sicknesses from childhood like mumps, measles, chicken pox, etc. to reoccurring yearly colds and flues, to more advanced cases like tumors, heart attacks, arthritis and cancers!! A gradual decline in the body begins in childhood really (although the person still grows and matures), as different parts and functions of the body are not properly fed and cleansed. As one body organ or part begins to decline or malfunction, other areas will begin to be affected. For instance, if you have a very heavy diet -- lots of meats, cheeses, pastas, breads, etc. most likely you will have constipation problems, which can lead to hemorrhoids, head aches, sluggishness, and at its worse colon cancer. Also, it strains the heart, as extra weight pulls down on the muscles and the chest lining and heart areas. Constipation could also cause a heart attack with the extra pressures in the body!

Diet suggestions:

A.   If you like the buffet restaurants, definitely pick one with a good, colorful and <u>fresh</u> salad bar with plenty of raw veggies. Most will have steam tables, with mashed and baked potatoes, corn, green beans, carrots, pinto beans, rice, hush puppies, cauliflower and broccoli, dressing (ask if meat juice free) and an assortment of breads. Leave the meat alone and if you really want to begin a better diet try one-half cooked food and one-half raw salad with all the colors available: carrots, cauliflower, broccoli, radishes, yellow squash, purple cabbage, etc. Don't be scared of the oil, use enough dressing to make it tasty, a wedge or two of lime or lemon is healthy and a splash or two of water balances it well.

If you are going to eat fruit or melon, eat them first along with plenty of water, and wait a few minutes before digging into the main course. Be sure to ask one of the chefs if in doubt of the ingredients used in their food preparation, especially if you are a Vegan (a meatless and dairyless vegetarian). Also, there are more delis and soup and salad places around these days, that have very good salad bars and baked potatoes, just stay away from the meats and cheeses.

B.   IHOP Pancake House has been an occasional treat for me in the past, I always have the country grain and nut pancake or waffles and bring my own 100% maple syrup, almond butter and coconut flakes. This way it is a bit more nutritious and heavy-duty for those active Saturdays. Also, they have tasty orange juice and coffee (try one-half cup of coffee with the rest the ice water, for a "tea-like coffee." You still get that coffee taste and kick and it's not so hard on your head and nerves, etc.)

C.   Some of your health food stores have a BarBQ Wheat Roast product that, along with some pickles and onions and a whole-wheat bun is a very tasty BarBQ sandwich. Also, the product called Vegitas exists, which looks and tastes similar to well-done roast beef. Put it on some multi-grain sandwich bread, with

Veganaise (dairyless mayonnaise), avocado and tomatoes, and it is quite tasty.

D.   Some of my recipes cooked and raw:

1. Breakfast

a. Wholegrain oatmeal – with soy protein powder, pure vanilla flavoring, raisins, walnuts or pecans (during winter when in season), margarine, Turbinado sugar or Sucinat (the most pure sugars available); nine grain toast, margarine, almond or cashew butter, and fruit sweetened preserves.

b. Quick and hearty coconut sandwich – nine grain bread toasted, margarine, and one-quarter grated fresh coconut or a dried packaged coconut (just put the margarine on the toasted bread and put the coconut in-between it and there is your sandwich), and vanilla or chocolate soy drink.

c. New Age Banana Pudding – Two medium to large bananas, some almond meal flour, and one heaping tablespoon of raw almond or cashew butter. Now with a fork, mash the bananas very well & blend the nut butter with the bananas. Blend one-half the almond flour with the almond butter/banana mixture. Sprinkle the other half of the almond flour on top for a crust.

d. Fruit salad: One handful each of red, green, and purple grapes; one handful each of raspberries, strawberries, and blackberries [or a relative & colorful combination], mint leaf (fresh if available or dry if not), a few shakes of pumpkin pie spice, some finely chopped ginger root, one-half lemon and one-half lime squeezed, and enough fresh orange juice to two-thirds cover ingredients. Stir well.

e. Fruit smoothie: One-third each of a red, green, and yellow apple, chopped up, four pitted prunes, a few shakes of pumpkin pie spice, a teaspoon of dried mint or a few fresh mint leaves and stems. Put all into a blender with unfiltered apple juice and blend well.

2. Lunch: (should be the largest meal of the day for active people).

a. Salad Number 1: Spinach, purple cabbage, carrots, cauliflower, broccoli, yellow squash, olives, tomatoes, sunflower seeds, croutons, dressing (add a few squeezes of lime, lemon or both and a splash of water).

b. <u>Salad Number 2</u> (good for blood, circulation, and immune system): Red, yellow, orange and green bell peppers, plenty of finely chopped garlic, grated raw beets, tomatoes, spinach, dressing as above, and cilantro.

c. <u>Salad Number 3</u>: Lettuce, purple cabbage, cucumbers, asparagus, okra, parsley, dressing as above.

3. <u>Supper</u>

a. In summer: Alternate watermelon and cantaloupe from time to time before the main course. Drink plenty of water with them and wait 15 minutes to allow digestion before further eating. (If the melon is eaten with or after the meal "gastric disturbance" is most likely to occur, as different food types take different enzymes to digest and when mixed incorrectly can react like baking soda and vinegar — causing gas, a bloated feeling, and perhaps fermentation of what you ate. There are many books available on food combining.)

(1) <u>Main course</u>: mashed avocado with cumin, cayenne, garlic and sea salt powders. Multigrain bread or tortilla chips if needed, with lettuce, tomato and dairyless dressing. One medium piece of carrot and celery. Water to drink and if Vegan or really ambitious and brave, some seaweed.

b. <u>Number two main course</u>: (Divine Muscle Infuser after a strong workout). <u>Coconut Shake</u>: one quarter piece of raw coconut grated, splash of vanilla, one tablespoon of almond butter, one handful of raw almonds, one or two shakes of sea salt, and one or two medjul dates. Blend well, add some ice and briefly blend again. Perhaps one piece of well done nine-grain toast with margarine also.

c. <u>Number three main course</u>: Before I began my raw food diet transition, I really enjoyed the Whole Foods Market BarBQ'd Wheat Roast; add some pickles, onions, on a whole wheat bun and everyone I turned on to it was really surprised. Some potato salad or curly fries mixes well also. Iced tea to drink.

<u>Note</u>: So, there are a few suggestions. There are countless books written with vegetarian recipes that warrant a beginners attention,

especially making the carnivorous to vegetarian transition! Strive for the best fuel for your body and satisfaction, and always use God as your Common Denominator in making your decisions in diet and otherwise.

Finally, to underscore my point about the traditional meat diet in relation to Karma or You Reap What You Sow! Have you ever seen the African Seringhetti documentaries on public television where the Lion devours the Zebra or the Wildebeast, then has to sleep for 20 hours while being constantly tormented by flies and fleas? It is not unlike human sluggishness after a heavy meat meal and their torment with mosquitoes and allergies, bothersome, right... think about it!! It's the Earth's Adaptation to Itself and in this way it is a never ending, self-perpetuating circle or cycle ... until we achieve meltdown or what I call **"Armageddon of the Darkness,"** or we change and create **"Armageddon of the Light"**! More on this in Chapter 11.

CHAPTER 3

Other Remedies

Pros and cons of the following alternative remedies:

Bee Venom Therapy - Sounds to me as if Bees are placed on the afflicted areas and made to sting the body part. Or perhaps, by some unique way, bee venom is extracted and then injected into the afflicted area... probably the former!

My conclusions: No pros at all, this is ridiculous! The cons - enduring the pain of the sting and possible trauma; possible side effects from the venom; again humankind enslaving another species of life for Frankensteinian Research! Let nature follow its own innate course, with occasional human guidance~

Magnets, etc. - I like this idea... As in my early years I was intrigued by them, not only how they magically attracted to each other, but even more so how they could also repel each other. I was mildly obsessed with trying to stick them together while opposing each other. The body has its own energy field they can be seen and measured with the proper equipment. Perhaps, if a video could be taken of the afflicted area, one could see what possible affect magnets might have upon it, as it is happening, especially with varying intensities of the magnetic force [use an electromagnet]. Now, in this idea it's energy affecting energy, which could be part of the curing process; but there is also the flesh, blood, and tissue aspect that has needs of another, but complementary form, as in diet!! No cons @ all. Copper bracelets had been the thing for a while, with testimonials galore! Perhaps, an interesting phenomena... we wear the metals and jewels of this Earth mainly as decorative adornments to compliment our attire and enhance our appearance, but in a paradoxical paradigm there lies Hidden Healing uses for these Elements also!

<u>Herbs -</u> Kava kava is a very good natural muscle relaxer and has a drowsy effect, so it's better to take in the evening somewhere near bedtime. Like I've said, if the muscles and associated parts are tense, the body will be more rigid and slower, and as one pushes through this extra resistance throughout the day, the various moving body parts begin to sustained minor injuries, which in time can become more serious! So, as some point muscle relaxers (preferably natural ones) can be used from time to time to help relax the body. Also, as in treating any sickness, anything to strengthen the immune system is vital, so here Echinacea & Goldenseal are a good combination to take! There are a multitude of Medicinal Herbs available in easy to take forms these days... do some research & consult an Herbologist! Also, if you're doing other complementary help aids & living a 'tight life', then you'll soon notice positive results in your Cure & Care for Arthritis. Remember, a more fluid & pain free body motion increases your quality of life... which you will feel until the day that you Meet your Maker!!

<u>Supplements</u> - Glucosamine and Chondroitin are obviously the first that come to mind... crushed animal bones and cartilage. I can see the understanding behind it, much like back in the fifties when I was made to eat beef liver, because it was good for my liver?? Folks, if the liver's function is to filter and purify the blood, why ingest something that might have toxic residue still in it?! But, the mainstream has already come to the rescue, saying that organ meats are now high in bad cholesterol. Now, a lot of people say that the glucosamine & chondroitin do work well for them, so perhaps in some unique way they are broken down and absorbed by the body or cause something else to affect the bones, joints, etc in a positive way. So, if something rather than nothing is working, keep doing it for now... but in the long run its shortcomings will most likely surface! Likewise, with calcium supplements, - how can a dead inorganic substance feed, heal, and cause to grow / repair a live organic body... that's not the way it works!!

<u>Massage and Chiropractic (balms - hot and cold)</u> -I believe I'd get a general consensus that these two therapies are very valuable in dealing with some of the pain of arthritis!! Keep in mind, that not too many decades ago, chiropractry was dismissed as quackery by the mainstream medical establishment! And, I'll remind you again with all the amazing medical apparati & incredible amounts of knowledge at

their fingertips... still no cures or even quantum leaps in the cure & prevention of arthritis!! Hippocrates, long ago said, " One day a Man's Food will be his Medicine."!! So, back to Massage & Chiropractry... first off massage generally is the manipulation of one's body by another, primarily with the hands, but also with the elbows and feet.

An adept Masseuse w/ strong & accurate hands can work the tension and energy blocks out of another's body & to a great degree alleviate a lot of the pain and stress! Also, a good Masseuse should listen to their patient for additional guidance! Massage is also very helpful before a chiropractic adjustment. The Chiropractor deals with the manipulation, adjustment, and alignment primarily of the bones and spinal vertebrae. Most often x-rays are administered to help diagnose and clarify the situation. Once one's body is out of proper skeletal alignment, a number of problems can occur that can cause aches and pains, which could be diagnosed as arthritis. So, I would definitely recommend Massage and Chiropractry in your Arthritis Healing Regimen, but do some research and find some good practitioners, as it makes all the difference! Additionally, there are balms and ointments that go hand in hand with massage and chiropractry, like tiger balm, bengay, or from the dollar store - muscle rub, it's as potent as any of them.

Yoga - a relatively passive form of stretching, posturing, and exercise brought to us from the Eastern Indian missionaries back in the 1960s... who also gifted us with the vegetarian ways and meditation!! In the last 40 years basic yoga has morphed into various forms and under American influence it's has become a multi $1,000,000,000 yearly enterprise!

Meditation - absolutely a high five! To put it simply meditation is relaxation of the body, mind, and spirit. In these stressed out critical days few really take 5 or 10 minutes a couple of times a day to decompress and recharge.!

Sit down in a quiet comfortable place, loosen the clothing, close the eyes, gently breathe, stop the mind chatter, keep stopping the mind chatter, relax the body, and keep doing all of these for a while. You'd be amazed at how much better yet feel, along with increased energy, and no negative side effects! When one doesn't take occasional breaks during the working hours to relax and ease stress, tension and stress can build up in the muscles and associated parts and cause stiffness, aches and pains, which could be construed as arthritis. But what is the

Usual MO - grabbing another coke, coffee, or energy drink or pill, sugar treat, alcohol, or whatever helps... with plenty of negative side effects!! For me 10 minutes works well - 5 minutes to settle down and 5 minutes of nirvana!

Different forms of meditation:

Mantra - probably one of the most common, transcendental meditation, being the most popular. I don't know too much about this but it seems that one takes a word or phrase to focus upon and if necessary to repeat, by which they are led into a deeper state of relaxation.

The Silva Method – I took it in the early 'roaring seventies', which was my first introduction into any meditation. It's based on achieving deeper levels of mind energy from Beta, to Alpha, to Theta, to Delta (most commonly - deep sleep). These levels are achieved by closing your eyes, doing some gentle deep breathing, while telling yourself to relax and go deeper, while counting down slowly from 10 to 1.

Buddhist sitting meditation -custom designed for the over active Western Mind... & one of my favorites, along with some of their teachings!

They remind me a lot of the American Indians... Very Down to Earth, & Be Here Now! The gist of it is you adapt a good sitting position on the floor sitting on a pillow. The exercise or meditation focuses on the simple fact of relaxed breathing and being present in the moment. The common tendency is to space out into mental tangents of thoughts or scenarios of something or many things. The crux is once you realize you're in some mind drama, you stop or conclude it and come back to the relaxed breath and present state of mind... it's harder than you think, but works amazingly well! I took a Buddhist meditation class in Austin, Texas and had a brilliant teacher named Beth... as I look back, my simple B.S. didn't impress her at all! I admired her Clarity and corresponding Spirit of Life, yet I guess something about me caused her to take me under her wing... just a little bit. Perhaps, it was a combination of being an aspiring vegetarian and having had some visionary experiences, which leaves its imprint upon you~ By the way, the 'Sits', as the Buddhist Meditations are called, are an hour-long... how long can you tread water...in other words, it's more difficult than one might think, but again very useful! A good book to read is "The Myth of Freedom" by Chogym Trungpa Rinpoche!

Wet / Dry Sauna and Whirlpool - I go to the gym at least twice a week, and while most are feverishly working out to varying degrees, perhaps less than 10% of the men and women take the relaxing and cleansing pleasures of the wet areas! Conversely, some regular older folks who routinely visit the wet area, amongst them maybe only 1/3 of them workout [perhaps something I don't realize yet, as @ some point, enough is enough, and they're in that sedentary stage of life when you've done your time and paid your dues]! Two important therapies however, that are missing from most modern day spas, are the cold plunge and inhalation room!

Transition from Mainstream to ½ Vegan and ½ Raw Diet - if one has a typical mainstream diet of meat and animal byproducts, flour products, mostly cooked veggies, and perhaps only 10% raw food, then your optimum physical years will be in your twenties. By the mid thirties the infamous midlife crisis has shown its frightful face as an impending reality! At 35, most have an extremely developed mentality and an evolving spirituality (which naturally comes as wisdom through the trials of life and can be enhanced with a deeper seeking in a myriad of ways). So, is it a Cruel Joke that God has played upon us... no, it's not Him, it's Us!! I said w/ a 'gut feeling' when I was 30 years old, that I was going to physically peak at 60 years old, and now at 57 years old I believe that even more so... but like the Pros say, 'It's harder & takes longer to get back in shape, & easier & shorter to get out of shape' !! To put it bluntly, the Methods of Healing in the Status Quo just aren't working as completely as we need, as we are still a very sick world!! The methods in place do support our current day and age, but at an ever increasing cost, as we seem to be on a slow downward spiral with a lot of torque and one that is gaining momentum! In other words, I believe there is a 'failsafe' point at which if we go by, the flow will not be able to be stopped!! The Christian Church calls this the inevitable Armageddon; I call it the 'Armageddon of the Darkness', which has an opposite which I call the "Armageddon of the Light'... though the Churches that Ascribe to the Former, have no Knowledge or Belief in the Latter - What a Shame!! The former being inevitable chaos, destruction, and sorrow; the latter, through becoming Responsible for the Sacredness of Life on Earth, Realizing the Human Commonality regardless of religion, nationality, race, age or gender;

and Realizing and Evolving into God's Family - as we come closer to God and Each Other, God comes closer to Us!!!

How this change from a animal based mainstream diet to a basic vegetarian, then vegan, then to a more raw food diet affects arthritis and any other disease, is simply that if meat and the byproducts were not designed by God our Creator for our Sustenance, and yet one consumes the meat and animal byproducts, the body will at some point, earlier than later, Begin to Malfunction! Eventually, these malfunctions began to turn into more serious maladies, sicknesses, and the common day diseases that we are all familiar with!!

In conclusion, 'What the world needs now, besides Love sweet Love, is Intelligent Complementary Medicine'!! I have said and I will say many times that I'm greatly appreciative of current day science and medicine, that keeps the status quo intact, but we desperately need some New Ideas, that are more simple to behold and innately basic to all life, harmony, evolution, and survival with a great vitality... **It's our Birthright!!**

CHAPTER 4

Will Pride and Greed Overcome Truth?

<u>Pride</u> - Pride is a tough question for anyone, when you think you are right or on the right path to discovery, you constantly reaffirm this with your thinking and it is also re-affirmed with what you choose to read and perhaps by friends or colleagues. Pride on one hand, is a worthy and deserved compliment to one's self when weighed with the balance of truth ... in other words your accomplishment that you feel good about is worthwhile to yourself and / or to others. On the other hand, pride is detrimental when one stubbornly holds on to lesser ideas or beliefs, supported by tradition or common thinking, just because they have the power or predominance to do so ... at that point I question their true intent!! It would seem if a problem has remained unsolved for ages, one would be open to most any idea that has a chance or could be intelligently argued! Obviously, the American Heart as a whole needs some work ... balanced with a little less overwork in other areas, like our jobs!!

History has proven resistant to change. Remember "Fulton's Folly?" Robert Fulton, the steamship inventor, was laughed at and ridiculed until he made it work!! With more cooperation and harmony it would have had happened much easier and sooner; with more resistance, maybe not at all!! Remember Noah ... well if there were ever "the days" these are them ... war, famine, drought, floods, earthquakes, tornadoes, hurricanes, disease, pestilence, civil disturbance, disharmony between races and sexes, etc., more and stronger than ever before!! More on this in Chapter 11.

<u>Greed</u> - Greed also enters in to our predicament in many cases! We seem to be evolving out of the "dark ages" and modern medicine and similar advances (painstakingly earned) have played a critical part in our survival! I am very grateful to this, because looking back I (and many others) probably would not be here today or in as good of health,

many thanks!! I am just trying to advance *"the cause,"* w/ this Special Knowledge I have learned, earned, and have been given in the last 30 years ... is not that what everyone wants??!!

Most Doctors and Scientists make a lot of money in the realms of our society and I am sure they enjoy this and are fairly secure in what their future holds, as compared with the more common working class America ... their Customer Base! I am all for the Capitalistic Notion, that is the driving force of American Production and Quality of Life - if one has the desire to do more or take greater risks than another, they should reap greater rewards! But to deny the much needed ideas of the *"alternative medicine and natural healing fields"* just to maintain your financial laurels, is definitely a form of greed, of dollars and power, and You Do Reap What You Sow... **no real cures for anything in sight**, a lot of sufferers – Drs. included!! Lobbyists, from a number of special interests, influence politicians and laws, which underscore this! On the other hand, right kinds of laws protect us from downright quackery, because a lot of people are naive about cures and with lack of real hope, will try almost anything: as with arthritis - bone meal and fish oil, shark cartilage, and numerous other supplements (including mega doses) and pharmaceutical pills with more and more of them notating medical disclaimers of possible side effects, while Reaping Billions of $$$'s, but certainly not worthy of Reaping That Kind of Payoff!! (Some of the above do affect the body to create or do something, but can not be used as cellular building blocks or detoxifiers, like the natural foods of the earth).

Also, bee string therapy, horse ligament, drugs which try to block nerve signals or pain to the brain, silicone lubrication injections directly into the joints, artificial hormone therapy and genetic engineering; mental affirmations denying existence of sickness and prayer only!! I think the current chemotherapy and radiation treatments should be suspended because of the severe side effects of being sick and nauseous and having your hair fall out ... some of these are Frankensteinian - it shows us our desperation and how far out of touch with ourselves we are! So, we need some kind of better balance in our laws to give good ideas a chance.

Our world is obviously off course: we are still constantly sick and disease ridden, with no major cures or advances, just more crutches and new diseases; catastrophic events are much more commonplace these days than most people think, because they are so busy they do not see the larger picture; countries at war with each other keep popping up, just as another conflict gets settled (or sort of); & the occurrence of violent events with school age youngsters is just crazy (not to mention the violence amongst the rest of us), & it underscores the need for a Balance of True Spiritual Education [not a Religion] versus Worker Education as we grow up!!! So much money is wasted in the world just to uphold the status quo! In a sense and unbeknownst to most, it is the ultimate greed!! Defense spending is one-third of our national budget (the world's largest) and probably a great share of most other countries, also ... <u>Spiritual Realization is the Key</u>, We are All God's (or whatever name you refer to about the Good, Holy, Creator of All) Family! Just think of the relief that True World Peace would mean!!! The defense industries could be subsidized (with defense spending savings) while they retool to other areas - like new forms of energy and transportation and other new discoveries ... there is much work to be done!!

However, before World Peace can be achieved it must pyramid down to peace within each country, state, city, community, neighborhood, school, church, jobs, friends, & family, all the way down to oneself!!! At this point, peace depends upon physical, mental, emotional and spiritual health! As I am dealing primarily with physical health, I will remind you of another tremendous national expenditure in **Health Care** (probably most people's greatest concern, & all over the National Agenda today)! As I have and will state many times the Mainstream's Meat and Dairy Diet is one of the main roots of sickness and disease (physically, mentally, emotionally, and spiritually). Begin to change this and the Real Healing with Begin. These days there are a multitude of transitional foods that will help you overcome "old favorites" until new and better habits are formed and a greater understanding is in place. And as with the defense industry, the meat and dairy industries (with health care savings subsidies) could retool into better and more organic farms, recycling and waste cleanup industries (we sure need that), and other areas. We need Revolutionary Change on our Earth soon!! Be intelligently open to it and look truly within yourself to see if greed is a factor in any resistance, and Pray for Guidance!

<u>Truth</u> - truth will overcome because it's Indelibly Inscribed in all of our Hearts and Souls! If everyone could see (or remember this), it would at least be an agreeable starting point! Though we are

constantly programmed in other ways: TV, movies, work, sports, entertainment, even most of our Churches do not Delve into Our Divinity - it is always something out there! We are stuck in the "Tower of Babel" mentality, too many people going in too many directions ... "Communication Being the Problem to the Answer" as a song once stated!! Not just the exchange of information, but how it is exchanged!

We have become too busy to learn to relate with each other for very long (a somewhat Dysfunctional World). At best, the busyness we get 'caught up' is creating the energy for change ... for the good or the bad?! I call the good the "Armageddon of the Light" and the bad the "Armageddon of the Darkness" - this is the bottom line, what it is all about, the Alpha and the Omega, our last chance; yet we are so shortsighted we do not see for very long and are soon back on our individual trains to oblivion, until something stops (our world) - like someone's death or some natural disaster, etc. More about this in Chapter 11.

One of my points with Truth is simply I believe God Ordained our Sustenance or Diet to be from the Earth as it Grows in the Seasons (as the seasons change so does our needs, though most eat the same year round). Most eat the neatly packaged, slaughtered animals and are removed from how that process actually evolves. The smell of driving within a few hundred yards of a slaughterhouse is indelibly inscribed in my mind and nostrils as the worst ever - I really did not think I could make it out of the area, it was sort of like being underwater and needing air ... and that was the first of three in a row!!! Plus the end costs of providing a pound of meat for food is ten times greater than food in a vegetarian's diet and the damage done to the earth (rain forest for grazing land, waste product disposal, water pollution, etc.) is more than that! Then you have the enormous costs of medical care throughout one's life due to an Improper Diet! The Impossible Idea of a quality and experience missed in one's life because of not feeling well and Reaching Possible Potentials! The Infinitesimal Damage done to all people and society through alcohol and drug abuse, crime, murder, war, and the Karma of the Mass Consciousness (hurricanes, droughts, earthquakes, famines, etc.); all with a major root in an improper diet (if you do not feel well, you cannot act well)!!

And I might add again, too much Worker Education and not enough True Spiritual Education, along w/ negative mass media input (garbage in, garbage out)!

In summary, Detrimental Pride can block or inhibit much needed change if one is in a position of power over others & abuses the power! This ties directly into Greed because if another idea or path, leads to better solutions, then the money will also follow!! I do not understand the Resistance to New Ideas in Ways of Thinking! Except that so many are living *on the edge* these days that the status quo is easier to accept than change. People have got about all they can handle and have little time to consider much else!! Well, Truth always wins out, but what we have to go through to get there can be either good or bad ... be intelligently open and **"Let the Truth set you Free!"**

CHAPTER 5

What this Could Mean For Pro Athletes and Sports

The team is moving along well, on paper all the voids are filled, the playoffs are on the horizon - then bam, bam, bam, a strain here, tendinitis there, a pulled hamstring over there ... well maybe the backups can hold on and maybe a trade before the deadline! Sound familiar, in Houston it sure does!

Pro athletes (as well as any exercise inclined person) could benefit enormously from my discoveries!! As much stress as they put their bodies under, pain and injuries are inevitable, in the status quo! Especially the partiers - the alcohol, drugs and other over indulgences, plus the pot of coffee the morning after really make them less supple, in the bones, muscles, joints, tendons, ligaments, tissue, etc., which count for most of the injuries. **While some injuries cannot be avoided, the team with less injuries will come out on top mostof the time!!** Also, I am sure that one of the most painful and stressful parts of athletics is morning after the game or contest or practice. Soreness, stiffness, aches and pains, and now you have to go out and prepare all over again! It takes a lot of time to warm and loosen up, not to mention the agony of doing so! This could be greatly reduced with putting to work some of my ideas. Individual accomplishments could also be greatly increased. Achieving greater heights in sports, could help eliminate the major problems of drug and alcohol abuse amongst athletes, along with a return to basic Harmony and Sanity. While this book is primarily about a Cure for Arthritis, you cannot achieve your maximum health and potential while still Ingesting the Slain Animals.

You will constantly feel an anxiety, caused by eating an animal's flesh, in which is entrapped the shock of its violent death - which affects the "predator" physically and emotionally. That is why I say a "Return to Basic Harmony and Sanity." Meat is not food, God did not ordain it that way, "Thou Shall Not Kill" ... animals are another form of life with their own sacred volition. Look deeply into their eyes sometimes, they are not so unlike us, just a different form!

To get to the point, improperly lubricated joints, muscles, etc. are much more prone to injuries and are also weaker and slower. Some analogies: do not clean and oil a rusty hinge and you can keep forcing a door to open and close, but eventually the rotating joints will become worn and loose and as its pressures change and the screws will loosen also; keep running your vehicle on low and dirty oil and your engine will use more oil and will wear out sooner; put off regular vehicle lubrication and you are in for some major front end repair and a rougher, riskier ride!! So, as an athlete, if you drink a couple of cups of coffee and only a little water and have mostly cooked or refined foods in the morning (even with no meat); have a mid-morning soft drink or one of those spacey looking pink, green, or blue energy drinks, or God knows what's in them energy bars; and for lunch a one pound of meat, cottage cheese, milk, salad (lettuce, tomato and a few carrot shreds), and a piece of fruit; and a cholesterol and sugar loaded mid-afternoon milkshake; and a couple of after work out brews with the guys & gals (this is during the week, the weekend could be much worse); and finally the evening meal, traditionally our largest, let's see - pizza, pasta, fish, chicken, cow, or pig and dessert ... a full stomach is not conducive to good rest not matter what you eat. Even with a moderate supper, eat at least three hours before bed, & you will sleep much better!

The athletes that can understand what I say and take the faith and diligence to try, will be the ones who become more injury free, who regain their careers, and the ones who rewrite the record books on a regular basis!! There is no reason why, even in the most strenuous sports of football, basketball, baseball, soccer, etc. where careers have usually peaked by their early 30's, that one cannot pay competitively well into @ least their 40's & maybe even 50's!!

As I have said and will say many times, "Use God as your Common Denominator" in anything you search for, wonder about, or try to achieve!! One of the greatest things you can realize is the existence of God & in that way Yourself!! Yet most are too busy to take the time and hence do not believe or even if they do believe, do not delve further and deeper to understand more and greater things ... it is not a priority! Tell me then, how does it all work? The day and night are guaranteed, as are the seasons; you eat your food, it's satisfying and your body takes care of the rest; plant the seed in the earth and it will produce what it came from! All in all we are really fairly intelligent, but we did not design the above and it did not just happen. A Source far greater than us put it all together and its Intriguing Mysteries keep pulling us forward towards the "Straight and Narrow Pathway." I choose to call the Source God, others call it Mohamed, Allah, Buddha, Jesus, Lord, Krishna, etc. However, many religions proclaim theirs as The Only True Way, & therein more Conflict is Born!!! Humanity writes the books trying to describe their own Stirring Spirit and Knowledge and while God inspired, none so far has Grasped the Whole Picture! Most religions have many great ideas and truths within them, so we should be sifting these out to develop a Truer Religion (that is how strong progress is gained in any other field)!! I believe there are "Absolute Truths" beyond our partial understanding, that is common to all!!

As more of us tune in to parts of this, "God's Family" will become Increasingly Manifest, rising out of its lost ways, sin, and apathy! With all this in perspective, there are two things I would like to see: one is more emphasis in the early years (5 to 18) on the many Good Spiritual Lessons available, to balance all the typical current Worker Education... this way the many juvenile problems we face could be solved and hence more efficient worker education and less resistance to it; the second is Sunday as a Holy Day (not a pro sports or a busy, busy day as it has become), but one in which we rest, pray, worship, relax, take in from creation, reflect on the past week, be with our family, etc. I still have a newspaper snippet on my frig in which the late Pope John Paul proclaims, "Sundays should be a Day for God, not Diversions like Sports & Entertainment!" {How True & Beneficial it could / should be!!} God Knows We Need a Rest!!

In summary, pro athletes are an amazing lot in their chosen fields of endeavor! Most of us are involved in some sports in growing up and many strive to become the best. As the best do rise above and go on to focus more of their lives in their chosen sport, they develop almost superhuman abilities that amaze, entertain and inspire us, the fans!! Sports create an arena in which we strive to develop our physical bodies primarily, but a true champion knows the mental, emotional and spiritual balancing aspects are the catalysts to his or her success!!

However, there is a growing imbalance in our needs to be entertained, have heroes to worship, and in some of the staggering amounts of money paid to athletes!! It's a game, business, and livelihood that is great to watch and play; & the best, like in any endeavor, should be paid well ... but it is not solving our world peace problems, not curing our diseases, or helping us find God or Ourselves as a Humanity!!

My purpose here is to help find our way back to a Greater Peace and Harmony for all! I believe some of my ideas could greatly help the pro athlete to excel better and longer than ever before and to become a more settled individual, through a more natural diet. Individuals and teams could be better balanced and less injury prone, specifically. More consistency and greater achievements could be had, with Camaraderie and Sportsmanship leading the way!! (I do not agree w/ the aspects of intentional or hard fouls in Pro Basketball ... if you get beat on a play you get beat, Take it Like a Man and strive to do better, not like a brat where injuries can result and tempers flare.) With a new stature of the game, the youth would be better inspired to emulate its players in better ways and the players would take a quantum leap towards being true heroes!! I am not saying there are not and have not been many great examples in the ranks of pro athletes, but as history far back will attest to, there have been countless bad and questionable examples even amongst the heroes and legends!! **Do not eat the animals or their byproducts and see what a difference it makes!!**

CHAPTER 6

What This Could Mean For Everyone Else

This is the main reason for my book!! At first, during my discovery, I did not know the seriousness of arthritis worldwide. An Arthritis Telethon one spring began my education: 50 [now 70] million sufferers in America, fourth leading cause of death, 100 different types (I believe all could be helped by my ideas), and $81,000,000 in funding in 1994, I believe. With eyes that are beginning to see, I see the afflicted as they move in stiffness, with limps, bent over to the side, with pain and many times shame and fear of becoming weaker and more susceptible to some of the lesser ways of society! Let me take a moment and address the shame ... it mostly exists because its "put upon" afflicted people (not only with arthritis but any sickness or shortcoming one may have) by others in critical judgment or oneupmanship, or to help them feel better @ another's expense!! If one has the time and energy to judge in that way, then you are helping to tear down humanity's harmony and not doing enough to help the Earth really survive for better days! "Judge and you will be judged," is very true, especially for Hypocrites - Traitors to the Real Cause... You Know Not What You Really Do, but you Will Be Held Accountable!!!

Hope is a vital stepping stone for our survival. & it goes hand and hand with its cousin Faith. Faith is belief in things yet unseen, but felt as true. Hope is a half step closer, it's like having a Glimpse of a Possibility and becoming Excited and Faithful. It's that Excitement, that creates the Energy, to take us from Here to There! Here being in the darkness about the Cause and Cure of Arthritis; of glimmers of hope from traditional ways, but not quite what was expected; and some time just plain resignation! There, being some things from God's Earth that work quickly and without Dangerous Side Effects, while making other changes that take longer. The Excitement is like a Rebirth that is Contagious, then Hope is Born Strong! God never meant for Life to be so Hard; but Life is to Live and Learn from, the Rules are In our Hearts and Minds to find by Searching and Understanding!!

I am 57 years old and have been a carpenter 38 of these years. I work out most every day (but never on Sunday, as it's a Day of Rest and Nourishment from God) and usually get about six hours of sleep a night. I can relate to the **"workers pain"** and discouragement that comes when just as you begin to master your work the physical body is breaking down, here and there! Just when the mind and wisdom is beginning to peak the physical body is hurting worse and in more and more places. I see this now more in others than feel it in myself, because I have taken steps into the Unknown with Faith in my Understanding and have begun a Healing and Maintenance Process on my Body. Although if I backslide at times, it does not take long for me to feel the pain, & longer to get back to where I was!! Our bodies (mental, physical, and spiritual) are meant to be finely tuned instruments, but most treat their houses, cars, and other things better than themselves! You have to deal with yourself and how you feel, in everything you do and in everyone you deal with ... why not go for it with yourself and give some new ideas a chance??!! You could get yourself on a path to feeling better than you have in years or ever before! If we just slow down a bit and focus on our basic health or how we feel (and those that depend on and are close to us), our lives in the world will work out better than most ever thought possible ...

Love One Another, might be Achievable in Reality more, as opposed to some Holy Meditative Scriptures! But, how can we love one another very well, if we do not love ourselves? Because we do not feel good and hence do not look our best, we must take a "Time Out" and Begin our Healing Processes! It does take a while to settle down, diagnose, and figure out our Healing Processes. The **"RedCross"** gave me an extremely important insight once in something I read that they printed, it was something to the effect that *'In order to begin the healing process, one must not deny their sickness or ill feelings'* !! And I expand - be who you are, how you feel [but don't disrespect others], right here, right now, without the subtle masks, illusions, egos or whatever you want to call them ... Be in Truth and the Truth Will Begin to Set You Free!

In the next chapter I will give a basic Overview of my Cure that I believe would offer significant help to most anyone with some Form of Arthritis. I'll go into specific details in what I think will greatly help and in many cases completely cure (unless you start backsliding) some forms of arthritis that I understand. Like I said, I **think All Forms of Arthritis have Many Parallels that would respond similarly under the same treatments!!** You have to begin the healing process and get into it a bit, before you will know the next step in healing or undoing what you've created! I made the discovery over twenty years ago and know it works, but I have not had the time, resources, cooperation, or dollars to research arthritis in all of its forms. I once belonged to the Arthritis Foundation for four years and have written countless letters to them without a single response ... just letters from them asking for donations. **Thereis not enough money in all of the world that would help in the directions in which they search!!!**

But they already have a Great Network setup, along w/ offering many good & helpful ideas for those afflicted, & of course a support system... so let's not waste time 're-inventing the wheel', but work more in a complimentary way!!!

CHAPTER 7

The Cure: 1/2 Diet and 1/2 Habits

<u>So, the lubricating foods.</u> Lubricate [Webster's] - a substance, as oil or grease, for lessening friction, especially in the working parts of a mechanism. Concerning ones bodily joints, there is a natural lubricating fluid called synovial fluid that is supposed to exist between the cartilage cushionings on each of the end of the bones in a joint. It is my belief that through primarily an improper diet that this lubricating fluid is not replaced through the years of wear and tear on the body, and at some point in time begins to wear thin, the warning pains ensue, and arthritis occurs!

Let me go back in time 22 years ago to the point of my discovery and my assumptions at that time that eventually evolved into my discoveries and this book. It was 1987, just outside of Trinity, Texas in a subdivision called Pinecrest, which my father, Ernest Burge, had helped develop back in the early, **'Roaring 70's'**!! I was taking a 2 mile run one afternoon and notice that I had some upper back shoulder and neck pain and stiffness, that was bothersome. As soon as I reached the halfway point, I would stop and after a short rest due 50 marine corps push ups (which I can still do today and probably 10 or 20 more if I needed to)! *** I gave some thought to the pains, as I twisted my neck and rotated my shoulders to help work out the stiffness. I had been a vegetarian since 1980 and through my new Paradigmatic Journey, which began in the mid 1960's, I had already begun to see the World in a Different Way than most people in the mainstream.

So, the first thought, without the blink of an eye, was what kind of foods could Lubricate the Body from Within?! That was the Assumption, on the Idea that God [or buy whatever name one has learned to call the Good and Omnipotent Creator of All... it's the same for all of us folks, we only separate ourselves with our thinking and programming, and actions] created the Foods of Nature in a nonviolent way, to feed, nourish, and sustain us. So, if we develop physical ailments, primarily the problem and solutions lie within our Diet and Habits!! I began thinking about possible lubricating foods, and being mechanically inclined and knowing the value of proper lubrication, visualized oily things or foods with a slippery viscosity or make up. Of course, vegetable oils, the various seasonal nuts, avocados, bananas, and then the most special one, OKRA!! I have no idea why I thought of Okra, as I had rarely eaten it... perhaps the Spirit, seeing I was on the right track, planted that one, so I could get a move on! *** I finished my 2-mile run and that evening went to the grocery store to collect my lubricating foods. On returning, the supper that evening consisted of avocado, okra, and a salad. I cut the okra up, discarding the head & tip, and cooked it while putting the knife that I used in the hot soapy dishwater. I ate my supper and soon after washed the dishes. I had developed a habit of washing the silverware with my fingers, that way I could feel when they were clean. Now hear this - when I picked up the knife that I cut the okra with and begin to feel / clean it with my fingers, it amazingly still had the okra sliminess attached to it... after 30 minutes in the hot soapy dishwater!! This Phenomena, really caught my attention and over the next two days I ate 10 pieces of okra twice a day. I went running again three days later and had sort of forgotten about my test and... perhaps I believed, but didn't really believe~ So, about ½ way into run, I remembered my test, did a quick body check, and viola - no pain or stiffness, just Fluidity of Motion!!! At that point **'a little light'** came on in my head and I said out loud, "Alright, I really have something here!!"

Again, the year was 1987, and over the next six years or so I would usually eat the okra @ least once a week. But to further test my 'Lubricating Foods Theory', when I got what I call the Arthritis Aches, I would double up on the okra [though other cravings suggested things more tasty to me in those days], & tighten up on my few remaining less than great habits I had in those days! How would I, or you, ever know if you didn't give it a good trial / try... Intelligence, Faith, and Willpower!!! Also, I have found out through Living Experience, that habits like the alcohol, smoking, and too much coffee and soda water can set off the Arthritis Aches by dehydrating the inner body, and also these habits follow the Law of Diminishing Returns as far as Benefits and Detriments!!

In either 1993 or 94, one Sunday afternoon, I just happened to tune into an Arthritis Telethon on TV. I was amazed at the amounts of money that the different pharmaceutical companies contributed to the foundation for research!! Also the general public contributed to the foundation and in that year the grand total was $81,000,000!! That really got my attention and it was at that point I decided to write my book, after naively but bravely calling into the Telethon to exclaim that I had a Cure for Arthritis, to which one of the operators replied, " Oh, that's great, and how much would you like to donate?!!" So, one Saturday afternoon I went to Herman Park to painstakingly begin to write the first book and after 3 hours of huffing and puffing I had about 15 chapters pretty much named and a few notes or " core thoughts" on each (core thoughts was one of my high school English teachers favorite terms - Mrs. Mary Grace Dent of Robert E. Lee High School - Houston, Texas 1970... Thank you so much for teaching me how to write)!!! As time went on though, the writing became easier, although keeping things in context was a constant challenge!

Many times I got on a roll with it by doing some writing early in the morning before work, during lunch time, and again late at night!! But, as is common for many in life, occasional indulgences put out the fire @ times! However, I never lost Faith in my Idea and knew that I had something very Valuable for Humanity!! So, through the rest of the 1990's I developed enough control to immediately go to the okra when the Arthritis Aches struck, which for me was usually in the morning. So, I'd eat 15 pieces for lunch along with my salad and by late that afternoon when I went to work out I already felt the soothing lubrication, simple as that that!! God didn't make Our World to be Impossibly Hard, but to be understood in ways of Common Sense and a Deeper Heart~

As a note, although I've been focusing mostly on okra here, some other good lubricating foods are - bananas, avocados, nuts in season, any liquid oil and any other Vegan related substance that would tend to reduce the inner frictions of the body! In the year 2000 a Quantum Leap idea came to me in a way that I termed, an "Okra Infusion" - 15 pieces of all okra with a salad dressing, without anything else to eat along with it, that way it would be more quickly and abundantly disbursed throughout the body... and sure enough it was!! Here's another good therapy and arthritis treatment - a one-day water fast, is an amazing, though fairly tough, healing process!! It re-hydrates the body tissues and dissolves painful and toxic crystals that can accumulate in the muscles, bones, and related tissue is, due to poor diet and habits, & not enough water! After the fast, double up on the okra for a few days, say 10 raw pieces for lunch and then some other food and then ½ raw and ½ lightly cooked or steamed okra for the evening meal. Additionally, eat at least one piece of raw celery for lunch and dinner as it's very high in 'real calcium' which are the building blocks of the bones, sinews, and related (I call Celery a Structural Food) and this is just as important as the lubricating foods, for it helps to rebuild the already weak bones, etc!! By the way, celery, according to modern science, is very high in calcium and sodium which most know is good for building the bones; as opposed to the common programmed idea that cow's milk builds strong bones... Cow's milk is for their Calves, simple as that - common sense!! Another important note here: if one's Digestion, Assimilation, and Elimination are not working properly these areas will need some cleansing, etc before much other progress with healing the body can be had!!

Well guys, I did my part within the first 10 years, I have written enough of the book and Empirically Perfected the Process, and in vain contacted at least 50 American Publishers and Agents to get these works published (along with many possible Benefactors); along with contacting several branches of the Arthritis Foundation, including the one in my Houston Hometown, and the NIH (which greatly funds the Arthritis Foundation), and a multitude of other relevant foundations... All to no avail!! Stubbornness to Change pervades the History Books, & is Alive & Well & Kickin right Here & Now... I'm sorry to say - but not as sorry as the Hurting Ones~

In summation, the physical body is like a machine in that it needs proper fuel and lubrication [lubricate -Webster's - a substance, as oil or grease, for lessening friction, especially in the working parts of the mechanism] to operate at peak efficiency, and unlike machines - in a relative comfort! So, I urge you to look at the Real Predicaments we face these days - we're physically a very sick and weaker world, and even with the amazing and hard earned Miracles of Modern Medicine & Science, our Disease, Ailments, and Stress are taking a tremendous toll upon the Peoples of our Earth and are a big factor in our Myriad of other Problems, simply as a result of the repercussions of being physically far below our best, quite a bit due to our Poor Diet &

Habits!! We still have time, as we're still here with a stable enough status quo~ But, as any Worldly enough Person can see, with the general state of things that we don't have an unlimited amount of time, as we come closer to the Fail Safe Point!! God Bless Us All and help us take Responsibility for Ourselves, our Earth our Home, and Each Other!!!

CHAPTER 8

The Arthritis Foundation 1948 - 2009 and $400,000,000 - Where They Stand

The mission of the Arthritis Foundation is to improve lives through leadership in the prevention, control and cure of arthritis and related diseases. The Arthritis Foundation pursues its mission through a focus on research, public health and public policy.

My point here is not overly criticize or make wrong the Arthritis Foundation, and other Health Establishments of the Mainstream! As I have said and will say many times, they can take you apart and put you back together, along with stabilizing you with their medicines, and for that I am very thankful!! But to state the facts, & point out some of the errors or limitations in their thinking and approaches; & to add some of my hard earned Knowledge and Wisdom, gleaned from 40 years of Research and Wonderment at our Myriad of Serious Health Problems on Planet Earth!! **The Bottom Line is to find the Answers for the Cure... Right?!**

It would be foolish, and a waste of Time & Energy to try and Reinvent the Wheel!! The Arthritis Foundation is a widely and deeply established institution, that has served a great purpose in trying to understand and cure arthritis, along with helping multitudes of people with arthritis to cope, get better, and have hope!! However, I belonged to the Arthritis Foundation from 1994 - 1998 as I was evolving my own Paradigmatic Discovery.

I contacted them, their affiliates and the existing chairs here in Houston dozens of times and not one reply, only more donation request letters!! I recently rejoined the Arthritis Foundation to see where it stands today, as talk of this DNA - Medicine [Denosumab from Amgen being the latest] and a deluge of serious and sometimes fatal side effects of current popular Arthritis Drugs [Vioxx, Clebrex, & Bextra] concerns me!!

The following are excerpts of interesting articles from **'Arthritis Today'** , the premier magazine of the Arthritis Foundation. A few from the late 1990's and some current ones, followed by my comments, along with a few interspersed in their article. God Speed!!

Calcium and Kids ['Arthritis Today' July - August 1997]

Calcium is of great importance during the rapid growth of childhood, we can all agree upon that! But, as for the all important sources of Calcium here's what they recommend & I mostly disagree: dairy products (the only reason a cow has milk is for her calf - common sense); seeds and nuts (OK) ; fortified (with chemicals from where?) bread and cereal, and orange juice [OK with me, especially fresh squeezed, or @ least 'not from concentrate'].

We are the only Species on Planet Earth that takes another's species milk (meant only for their young) and eggs (an egg is an egg with a purpose, not unlike the human female egg - catch my drift?) to supplement our diet and we call them **"food"**...it's ridiculous, but the programming is deep, and hard to break, and has the Fear Stigma of - where will I get my Calcium and Protein... " drink milk for strong bones" and "eat meat for protein"!!

Nowhere is Celery mentioned, which is very high in Calcium and Sodium 2 major elements of Bones and also Ligaments, Tendons, and Cartilage!! And as an added benefit - definitely no cholesterol, a lot of roughage, easy to digest, assimilate, and eliminate, and good for the teeth just by chewing! There's just something about "celery and bones" though~

So, **"Get Celery and Lose Arthritis"**

The Knee ['Arthritis Today' September - October 1997]

The artists 'knee conception' is the best I've ever seen as it gives a good idea of what the inner workings of the knee really look like! Other than injury, there are many reasons for knee problems, and one of the most common is having to support too much weight, as in one being overweight, a very common problem in the U.S. , for a Myriad of Reasons!!

The *Synovium*, encapsulates the knee joints and secretes lubricating substances [synovial fluid] that create a frictionless film between the cartilage of the two bones, sort of like the front end suspension joints of an auto. As long as they are greased up well and in good shape, there is the ease of operation and no problem... but once there is metal to metal, or cartilage to cartilage, and then bone to bone, then Arthritis has stricken!! There's many lubricating food types that I've mentioned in Chapter 8, but **Okra** is by far the best (the difference between axle grease and oil, longer lasting and more durable) !! However, if ones digestion, assimilation, and elimination are not in good working condition, or if one's body is very toxic or broken down, the results will be much less, until one begins a Serious Healing Regimen!!

In Mainstream Medicine, many times a Synovectomy Procedure is performed, which is the removal of the thickened joint membrane called the Synovium, that causes damage to joints... what does this thickened joint membrane consist of - I'd say a really toxic and clogged up waste product affected tissue!

While my studies have dealt more with Osteoarthritis than with Rheumatoid Arthritis, the pain and inflammation of rheumatoid arthritis is sometimes caused by what they call Gout - I call it Extreme Toxicity from an Abusive & Improper Diet (and associated habits) and a poor and probably clogged up elimination system (kidneys and colon)!! Inflammation and Pain are Warning Signs - don't try to block them too much, but do Something Smarter!!

So, very often the mainstream solution is various types of surgery from arthroscopic [cleaning up debris], all the way to a total joint replacement... amazing, but tragic, **simply because ofthe Mainstream's Lack of True Understanding of a Proper Diet and where God our Creator fits into the picture** (I call Him the Common Denominator) with the Creation of Nature and the Natural Foods thereof and the Extreme Intelligence behind them!!!

So in a nutshell, we enter this world as a new creation and are given our start by our Parents Genetics & Health. But even in the womb of our mother, we are nourished by the tradition and whims of her diet, and once birthed into the world still mostly under these auspices till weaned from her breast!

So, even from conception; birth; being weaned; childhood under the auspices of family, peers and tradition; until we're all on our own, we are and have become much less than we could be... Sad, but True!! But, take Hope and Faith w/ This and Begin to Change and See!**A Subconscious Motto**..."I'll try and do anything, just don't mess with my diet, too much!!"

A Cartilage Substitute ['Arthritis Today' March-April 1998, page 19]

[Osteoporosis is the 'wear and tear' disease.]

The 'Advanced Biosurfaces' company is out of the Minnesota has come up with and tested this process: doing an arthroscopic surgery on the knees of sheep (somehow don't think the sheep had arthritis or damaged cartilage, so perhaps they're scraping away perfectly good cartilage... poor sheep] to scrape 'damaged' cartilage from the bone surface and apply a liquid polyurethane (you know, like brushing on for wood finish?? They didn't specify, but I'd think it'd be highly toxic, must be a water based] to these areas, which sets up very quickly to "restore the joints surface"! How about **"Poly Teflon"**~

So, as this was 10 years ago, I Googled "Advanced Biosurfaces" and ran into a few Animal Exploitation Websites (good for them... This Frankensteinen Research has got to stop, along with the toxic and disease causing diet the mainstream stubbornly has and Reaps the Karma Thereof!! Anyway, the public wasn't buying that idea - I wonder why?! In 2004 they developed a polymer cartilage for implantation... In extreme cases (and there are a lot of them) this may be viable, so good luck to them in that realm!

Also, a drug called Alendronate is being prescribed touting its claim that it bonds to the mineral in bone, reducing the activity of cells that normally break down the bone and allowing more bone to form. They say it could take 3 years of use to make significant changes in bone density or fracture risk... You cannot create live Organic Material, i.e. Bones, from inorganic medicine! You might be able to stimulate this or that to temporarily produce more, but without proper nutrition and building blocks it cannot happen for very long or well, not to mention possible side effects! Also there is no estimated cost listed for

Alendronate?? I stopped my search there, as you catch my drift & My Time is Anxious!!

Celery for the Bones, Ligaments, Tendons and the like; Okra for Lubrication or to fill back up the Synovial Fluid!! This is just part of the answer though, as one's body must be properly hydrated, and very importantly w/ such a Predominant Poor Diet in this Country (and World) a lot of cleansing must accompany the changes in Diet and Habit... Good Luck, Buena Suerte, and Start Changing for the Better!!!

Glucosamine and Chondroitin   ['Arthritis Today' Sept. - October 1998, pg 46]

Glucosamine and Chondroitin and are natural substances found within the body that are essential to the metabolism of cartilage... so hence the wannabe names~ Touted as cures for osteoarthritis, the supplements are formulated from: crab, lobster, and shrimp shells for glucosamine; and from cattle trachea for chondroitin! I've also heard that some comes from shark cartilage. It reminds me of a time back in the 1950s and early 60's when eating beef liver was supposed to be good for your liver... anybody remember that?! That and other organ meat foods were later debunked as high in bad cholesterol. Bottom line comes to a simple, yet juvenile association of like body parts between different species, and a naive common sense, but primitively understandable!

There has been many cases of reported relief from a multitude of partakers and those who swear by them! Perhaps they got lucky, and it does offer some minor relief & stability, whether real or imagined, but it's just another Panacea... that keeps the masses astray and is reaping billions of dollars once again for the pharmaceutical companies, etc.!!

If you really want some relief from the pain and suffering, begin a steady intake of Celery - one stalk with some salad dressing or hot sauce, and some chips or peanut butter (the old favorite) for lunch and one for supper, along with some okra infusions (lunch only, so it has the rest of the day to work into your body and go where needed) once a week three days in a row (10 - 15 pieces raw or lightly cooked) or every other day for two weeks!!

If you eat it Raw (the best: live food and enzymes to a live body) cut the tips and top off and chew 2 to 3 medium size pieces at a time and if needed add a teaspoon of your favorite salad dressing halfway into chewing your bite.

For lightly cooked okra: just cover the okra with water and a little bit of oil and soy sauce, some herbs and spices, and bring to a gentle boil. Once tender to the touch of a fork, take from the burner and add in some precut tomatoes, onions, and parsley or cilantro to help it cool, as they all meld together... be sure and also drink the 'slimy broth'! Additionally, w/ either raw or cooked okra [infusion] eat it by itself [10–15 pieces], as nothing else gets in the way or lessens the impact or speed to the painful areas!!

Color your plate ['Arthritis Today' March - April 2009, pg 31]

Vibrantly colored fruits and veggies contain high levels of phytonutrients (that's a new word... but leave it to science to further complicate the dictionary). " The more colors you eat at once the more powerful it is," says Dr. Stephen Pratt. He's heading in a good direction, but has left out an important point... don't mix your fruit and veggies, unless you want indigestion, gas, and lesser results!! In this article they've listed several different colors and associated foods with similar colors and what vitamin or mineral these foods are high in and what subsequent functional advantage they have for one's body. Science needs $1,000,000 electron microscope to investigate the atomic structure of foods in order to get a clue as to their purpose for the human body!

However, a good set of eyes, an intelligent mind, and a spiritual based heart shows you something else to be more obvious and exact!! More on that in my next book~

Nourished by Nature ["Arthritis Today' supplement guide Oct. 2009, pg 70]

<u>25 natural products for pain and inflammation -</u>

Finally, and at long last modern science is giving some 'reluctant credence' to some alternative or natural products... because 1/2 of America has been vigilantly seeking alternative remedies in increasing numbers the last few decades!!

"For mild osteoarthritis or rheumatoid arthritis, some supplements in the right doses can be of great help for treatment and decrease overall treatment cost, as well as possible side effects," says Dr. James McCoy (wasn't he in Star Trek??) a member of the Arthritis Today medical advisory board.

Here's a few to consider - their reasons and my comments:

Avocado oil extract -slows down the body's creation of inflammatory chemicals (why would the body do that, now?] Me - and it has a little oil lubrication, so less friction and thereby less inflammation... but eat the whole avocado instead.

Black currant oil - the oil of the seed contains 15 - 20% gamma-linolenicacid [GLA]. The body uses GLA to make chemicals that reduce inflammation, a lack of GLA may contribute to bone loss. Me - again I believe inflammation comes as a secondary warning sign after initial pain signals are ignored or nothing can be done about it, simply because of an Improper Diet and subsequent Habits. The mainstream diet does a poor job of providing proper sustenance and building materials to maintain a healthy body with consistent energy, and being able to properly cleanse and repair as needed!!

Several Herbs are mentioned, & along with others that have been around for eons and in all cultures around our Earth, that are very beneficial!! I know a good bit about Herbs, but would recommend seeing 2 or 3 Herbalists dedicated in that field, for advice and guidance! Also, try and find a good or book or two and educate yourself.

MSM Methylsulfonylmethane - that name enough (21 letters) should let you know it's not a natural product... they slipped that one in there - the sneaks! It's a sulfur product that helps the body form connective tissue & reduce nerve impulses that transmit pain. Me - a better way to 'form better connective tissue and reduce pain', is from new tissue formation and better lubrication in only 10 letters - okra / celery ; add water and make it 15 letters - with no side effects unlike MSN !!

SAM-e it's a synthetic form of a natural occurring chemical in the body which claims to treat stiffness, pain and joint swelling, improve mobility, rebuilds cartilage and eases symptoms of osteoarthritis. An anti inflammatory and analgesic, with the similar stomach irritation side effects as MSM.

<u>Me</u> - by now, you should know my agenda... so wholeheartedly begin to develop a much better diet headed in the Vegetarian / Vegan direction with a lot of emphasis on more Raw Food, and as always Celery and Okra and more Water, along with more cleansing foods and regimens [there's a lot of very good books about Healing Regimens and Fasting and Colonic Irrigations [closed system type, according to Bertha Canales of Houston, Tx.]... Go for it, and you'll soon be glad you did!!!]

<u>The Real Arthritis Diet</u> ['Arthritis Today' - Just Diagnosed pg 11]

"Arthritis diets are a dime a dozen. But can your menu really cause or cure arthritis? Probably not. **[I beg to differ and will vehemently so!!]** Only Gout a form of arthritis cause by uric acid buildup (a meat by product, by the way!) has a specific food / arthritis connection. Experts recommend a healthy balance of foods for a proper diet. Go for whole foods - fruits, veggies, whole grains... the less processed the better! Research shows that diets rich in nutrients can help arthritis and general health:

<u>Omega three fatty acids</u> - (how can an acid be fatty?) Fish.

<u>Vitamin D</u> - eggs; fortified breads, cereals, and milk.

<u>Vitamin C</u> - berries and citrus fruits. [I'll only agree w/ this]

<u>Me</u> - This just underscores the vast difference w/ mine & the understanding of the Arthritis Foundation, along w/ General Mainstream Practitioners, that the only thing we put into our body has little or nothing to do with its proper function or malfunction as pertaining to Arthritis [& probably most other sickness and disease]... **Utterly Ridiculous!!! I say it has everything to do with it!!!**

They have had more than enough time and money... Let's try some Other Ideas... unless you're not in enough pain??!!

Science without Religion is Lame ; Religion without Science is Blind~ Albert Einstein

<u>Understanding</u> = Health Formula... Michael Burge 10-8-2009

God

CHAPTER 9

I Need Grass Roots Funding Support

In the mid-90's I began writing about My Discovery - 30 minutes in the morning, before work at 7:00; 30 minutes during lunch, and 30 minutes before I went to bed at midnight… for quite awhile, as writing a book was totally new to me, but I give a Ton of Thanks to my High School English teacher Mary Grace Dent, who instilled in me the basics w/ a Fiery Resolve!! I have known about the okra, etc. effect for 22 years and it alone could help half the Arthritis Afflicted People, if not more. I solicited funds during the first year of my writing and collected $109!! I did my carpentry construction work 8 - 12 hours a day, but never on Sunday, and my creative energies became greatly drained, not to mention my spirit!! Yet as I began to write the words flowed, moved by the Need and My Desire! With sufficient monetary support I could of finished writing and had this book published years ago & have gotten this valuable information to the people!! Seminars still could be given and of course studies and tests by the Established Medical Authorities!! I would welcome this, Cooperation with Alternative Medicine needs to be established more to Sustain Our Future. The Arthritis Foundation already has a great network set up … but some of the Main Resistance lies in Chapter 4. If we do not make some major changes soon, in a lot of areas, the world will continue to suffer for it!! I wonder how much money is spent on health care every year?! Astronomical amounts, I am sure! We make life ten times harder because of our basic Ignorance and Stubbornness, and lack of Real & Deeper Camaraderie amongst the Human Family!! Life for many, is what I call trudgery - going through the motions without much sustaining hope… a Tragedy!!

We have a minuscule possible to really turn things around with some breakthroughs in Health and Nutrition like mine (more about that in Chapter 11), but without some Faith and Money … I do not know!! I have written countless Wealthy and Influential people, some of who think my writing is nice, **but avert the dollar issue!!** I spent several weeks doing library research on Texas Foundations when I was out of work at the end of 1996. I was surprised at the number of Foundations in Texas, especially Houston, and even more amazed at the Huge Amount of $$$'s they have!! I naively wrote 30 or so Foundations who fund under the headings Health, Medical Research, Specific Named Diseases, Diet and Nutrition, etc., and only received a couple of replies and no hope of money~ I have written several Arthritis Foundation's around the country, including the headquarters in Atlanta. Also, in my hometown during that time of Houston, I wrote the 16 Chairpersons on the Arthritis Foundation Board of Directors. No response, not even one, just letters requesting More Donations ... and I had belonged to the Arthritis Foundation for four years! I would think that in a "correct world" they would give anypractical idea a chance, with 50 million people afflicted and nearly $100,000,000 a year spent. They, like other scientists looking for the cure to Humanity's Myriad of Illnesses, continue to blame the causes on some germ, or gene, or unknown amoeba. The answers, like in many great things are simple, right in front of their noses (or mouths), but they cannot "See the Forest for the Trees"!! Finally, I wrote the National Institutes of Health, which greatly funds the Arthritis Foundation and sent them a preliminary overview of my discovery. They thought it was nice and would document it, but of course no dollars or further guidance! So, I appeal to those with Eyes that See, Really See our Human Worldly Situation! God did not design our bodies to break down just as our minds really mature and our spirits grow wise! But take a good look around and see through the Mist of Illusions at our Real Burdens!

I had a long term goal to have some of my knowledge out and working by the year 2000… it didn't happen though, @ no fault of my own, except that I couldn't Walk on Water!! So, at the start of 1999 I sold my pride and joy 1975 Corvette, and moved to my favorite Texas place, Austin - a very conducive place to writing, especially this type of book!! I lived off the Corvette $$$'s for 9 months, until my truck broke down & I had to go back to my carpentry work. I did complete 7 of 11 Chapters in typewritten form. My Format… taking my rough drafted notes, writing them out in long hand, taping them onto a cassette player, mailing them to my typist in Houston, who then typed them onto her computer while listening w/ headphones to the cassette tapes!! On subsequent trips to Houston, I would review & make corrections to the typewritten copies, & she would transmit this to the computer… & that's the way it was~

I have some valuable answers here & need financial support to put more of My Energy into this & help get it out, proven & established – it works people!!! This is just the tip of the iceberg, as you will see in the remaining chapters!

CHAPTER 10

Relation Of This Cure To Other Diseases

(Being a "lay person" in the Healing Fields, perhaps some of my terminology, definitions or examples are not perfect! However, I definitely believe I am close enough in my understanding and articulation to make my point very clearly understood!)

Disease is a disorder of the mind or body marked by definite symptoms (Webster's). I believe that basically any disease starts with one's Diet and Habits. Obviously, Genetics and Heredity gives us our Strengths and Weaknesses and if we would start early in a child's life working on the weaknesses instead of waiting for some sickness or disease to occur, life as we know it would take a quantum leap? Also, if parents would wait before creating a child, and work on their weaknesses until they are stronger or more balanced health, then their children would be much healthier!! Most likely @ some point in time, prospective parents begin to worry about even being able to have children!! Though I have seen some pretty healthy babies come from less than healthy parents ... we still have All the Grace in the World to solve our many problems, but no time to delay! Also, there are other factors such as Mental, Emotional, and Spiritual Problems that can have a tremendous influence on one's health, no matter how good of habits and diet one has ... but that is another book or readings that are pretty well covered by other writers. I would again add one bit of Holy Wisdom - We are All God's Family in our Deepest Sense, though we move too fast to take the time to realize, contemplate and readjust to this; like Jesus said Love One Another is the greatest Commandment of all ... until we settle down and find our True Nature, we will be lost and very problematic, & much less than we could be!!

So, the Relation of this Cure to other Diseases?! Take for example a relatively healthful baby in a middle class situation with a traditional lifestyle. I have seen so many little ones so congested they can hardly breathe ... it is no wonder because most nursing mothers have a very heavy congested diet: besides whatever meat, the extra dairy products recommended, the flour products in breads and pastas (add a little water to even whole wheat flour and rub it between your fingers and see how sticky it is - do you think it's much better once the body tries to completely break down the breads & pastas?). Probably with most nursing mothers not enough good water spaced throughout the day; and lack of at least one-half raw and one-half cooked food at each meal (with the cooked being fresh and seasonal as possible, and the raw being seasonal but not a mix of fruit and vegetables together, as they take different enzymes to digest and digest at different speeds and would cause indigestion, fermentation, etc.). Also most formulas have a lot of dairy and a wild assortment of vitamins and minerals and sweeteners that somehow nourish and sustain the baby, but sometimes make them go wild ... I have seen them walking back and forth, shaking hands and feet and bug-eyed, no wonder hyperactivity is so prevalent throughout childhood & beyond!! It can also lead to many emotional, mental and physical problems, not to mention the side effects from counteracting medicines. <u>Once again the problem with dairy is basically simple</u> - a cow's milk is meant for its calf, that is it, you do not cross species!

So, we have done it, that is why I think it and the absorption of milk from nursing mothers, baby foods, and eventual direct ingestion [along w/ associated meat products] causes childhood diseases like mumps, measles, chickenpox, etc.! They are the body's reaction, adaption to foods humans were never designed to eat!!! If this sounds strange or upsets you, then why have the answers not been found in all these years and with all the dollars spent?! I realize that most everyone is trying very hard in their lives and their schedules are very full! So the changes I mentioned in this book and their reasons may rock some of your foundations, which have been long and meticulously established. Try understanding these "new, old" ideas with an open mind, take it to prayer, have some faith and give it a chance! There are Paradigmatic... Seeing the Problems & Solutions from a different point of view!!

So, we survived childhood (those some do not or well enough) and enter our adolescent and puberty years. I remember mine and though I have countless fond memories and a really great family, I now focus on the negative aspects of sickness patterns and their probable causes. I remember the stomachaches and colds and sore throats - usually three or four per year, probably one per season. In particular I drank very little water in proportion to milk, 10% fruit juice, sodas, etc. Breakfast: refined oatmeal, margarine and white sugar, white toast, margarine and refined jelly; eggs cooked in Crisco, sausage or bacon, white toast, margarine and refined jelly; French toast (white bread dipped in egg, vanilla flavor, and white sugar combo). Lunch at school: meatloaf, creamed potato without skins or white rice, canned green beans or corn, and milk, and your typical other menus, though I hear they are a bit better now? If I brought my own lunch - two sandwiches white bread, mayo, cheese spread and hunks of lunch meat (the more, the better, the stronger I would be), chips and 10% fruit juice. (I always felt like going to sleep after eating lunch during school, I wonder why?)

After school snacks - at the golf course a Coke and candy bar and few sips of water here and there. Supper - meat, meat, meat, meat, meat (every meal) and supper traditionally largest meal of the day, no wonder I did not do homework well after supper - my mind was working on my stomach & My Fire was put out!. Again I am very thankful for my young life and all those who helped me along ... but we have some very serious problems and I believe I have a few important answers that will help solve them!

Here are a few of the Common Diseases and Illnesses that plague humanity and have so far eluded solution.

A. Common Cold - I laugh and helplessly shake my head at the TV commercials depicting people with runny noses, sneezing, and then Mom or Doc saying "Oh, you have a cold, we must stop that at once, here take this and this," ... did you ever stop to think that this is the way the body cleanses itself, by getting what we call 'sick'?! Instead of taking all of these medicines to dry up the cold, one should help the cleansing process along and let it run its course! I believe when the body heats up (a fever), it is the result of several things: the body's elimination system is plugged up - bowels from constipation; congested lungs and sinuses from dairy and heavy foods and not enough water; a general toxicity in the body; overwork and not enough rest! The first three relate directly to an improper diet. When the body heats up, a fever & a cold usually happen, as it is thinning down the congestion so it can be eliminated, hence runny noses, watery eyes, sneezing, &

fever etc. & then the suffering ensues! Allergies follow the same scenario ... why would anybody be allergic to the air and the common particles in it (dust from the air or from the dry grasses, plants, trees, or pollen, etc.)?

Now I am not talking about pollution, which is increasing in abundance, but even these in moderate levels should be easily handled by a healthy body! Those afflicted by allergies most likely could trace their roots to improper diet, definitely not enough water, not enough aerobic exercises and perhaps emotional blockages. Keep in mind everyone is different and each must carefully reverse and correct the Diet & Habits that led to their Predicament ... it is like working through a maze - carefully identifying the mistakes and making alterations then the next step will be presented (this is very important and something you cannot predict until you start unraveling one's patterns)! Lastly, without proper and complete cleansings which can include: stronger diets of cleansing foods - limes, lemons, ginger root, dry and fresh herbs, onion, garlic, jalapeno and cayenne peppers, etc.; plenty of water; a one-day juice fast, followed by a one-day water fast; enemas or colonic irrigations; saunas; and plenty of rest - a cold could turn into the flu or pneumonia, depending upon one's general health, strength and age.

B. Heart Attacks - the heart is essentially a pump pulling in revitalized blood and pushing it out into various parts of the body. When one of the arteries or veins or the heart itself becomes clogged up, the heart must work harder to eventually do less. This clogging process is widely associated with the over accumulation of unhealthy cholesterol from meat grease, cheese, too many heavy foods like breads and pastas (especially refined) and even too many salts and sugars (especially refined). After this constipated bowels (from the above-mentioned foods as sources of unhealthy cholesterol) and excess gas (from improper food combining and too many carbonated beverages) and one has greater enormous amount of pressure and stress upon the heart, not to mention many other organs!

Also, if elimination is blocked, digestion and assimilation are also affected thereby weakening the entire body from lack of proper nourishment and cleansing! With blocked bowels, heavy slow digesting foods, and large appetites, one most likely would develop a large mid-section, thereby further restricting heart expansion and contraction (and a major cause of mid and lower back problems). This heavy, improper diet also congests the lungs and the ability for strong, relaxed breath (an often overlooked area in the energy creation and circulation process). So taking into consideration any or all of the above examples, you can see how once again habits and diets directly affect a disease and in this case could cause a heart attack, the number one killer!

C. Cancer - I believe a lot of times it is not because the cancer is growing, but because an organ or tissue, or wherever a cancer is located, is <u>dying</u> from lack or nourishment and cleansing, so it appears to be growing! Other times, perhaps, it is a direct result of improper foods and additives never meant to be eaten, that causes a strange mutation called cancer. In either case, once again the big three - Digestion, Assimilation, and Elimination of Improper Foods is the Main Cause!

Most food eaten is cooked and hot when ingested and after eaten starts to cool inside the body (it also heats the body up a bit, so it is better in hot weather not to eat too much hot foods or beverages). With heavier foods, especially meats, cheeses, breads and pastas, they tend to thicken up upon cooling, take longer to digest, are harder to assimilate, and much harder to eliminate and generally begin to clog the body up! Hence the nourishing and cleansing processes begin to become inhibited and also the resulting congestion makes it harder to breathe clearly and strongly thereby reducing one's energy.

This starts in early childhood and as I have already stated is a root cause of colds, flu, fevers, headaches, stomach aches, and the like. As we grow older our diets and habits become more complicated and not as controlled! Add to this social pressures and work stress, and the "elixirs and potions" that are used to energize and relax us, and there begins the roots of major health problems! I will conclude my understanding of cancer with more detail of colon, lung, and brain cancer.

<u>Colon</u>: I believe the most common of all cancers and why not it begins in our largest indulgence – food. After the processing of clogging the bowels and periodic constipation has gone on for many years, diverticulitis or bowel pockets begin to occur (appendicitis can be a

direct result of this also). Keep in mind, the actual colon tissue has become weakened because of poor nutrition and add to this the bowel pockets and there you have the beginnings of cancers and tumors (hardened pus pockets from infected tears or wounds due to old and crusted fecal matter). It is not pleasant to talk or read about, but ask an experienced colonic irrigationist, fasting practitioner, urologist, or surgeon, and some can relate tales of five, ten, 15 or more pounds of this unelimated waste matter ... sounds unbelievable, but now you may start to see what I am saying, it is very simple!

Lung (and throat): With this cancer probably the first thing that comes to mind is smoking not just of tobacco, but marijuana, crack cocaine, and any other smokable substance (I have lost several close friends and acquaintances to this preventable disease). The lungs are meant for breathing air and oxygenating and energizing the body! While the above smokings are obvious causes of lung cancer, I believe that congested lungs from improper diet is also a major factor, as well as overeating, because the lungs do not have enough to expand and are not strong enough to lift the diaphragm, in which the stomach is encased.

A yoga instructor once stated that most people need to get in touch with their breathing more and through breathing exercises, lift their lungs out of their stomachs - how true that is! So, if you do not use something as strongly designed, it tends to atrophy and grow weak and become more susceptible to disease. An overlooked factor is overindulgence in strong beverages like hot coffee and alcohol, which directly come in contact with the throat and in time can dry out and make it brittle. Also the fumes, which carry some moisture, can directly affect the lungs with a burning sensation, like indigestion, which also can occur. I have not mentioned yet another well known factor - air pollution ... our body health and earth health go hand in hand, once we really begin to Heal Ourselves, we begin to know better than Pollute Our Earth! So, the combination of some or all of the aforementioned situations can play a major role in the development of lung or throat cancer.

Brain - as with lungs any smoking can adversely affect the brain and probably more so, because the head is the highest part of the body and any circulation restriction would affect it first. The brain needs plenty of oxygen to function properly and any restrictions of oxygen creates more tension and stress as one navigates their way through these chaotic times! ("brain breathing" strongly and directly through the nose, helps energize, oxygenate and relax this all important organ.) Tension and stress, in an organ, definitely blocks the energy flow and can be part of the problem. Also constipation can cause headaches and limit the amount of bodily nutrition to the brain - the nutrition being already depleted because of a poor diet!

Another important factor is learning to turn off the mind chatter, worry, etc. which constantly affects most people, and learn to relax!! This is brought to light in my studies of Yoga and Buddhism, which I am very grateful!

Stop and smell the roses, be here now, stop the constant self-reflection for a while, stop your false ego, or whatever else is leading you astray, and realize the Preciousness of Your Life and Others ... the way we behave sometimes is a Tragic Shame!!!

D. AIDS: I will be brief and to the point here. AIDS is predominantly a homosexual disease (more homosexuals have it than heterosexuals) and that alone should be enough to let anyone know the right or wrong of homosexuality! However, many heterosexual people have AIDS also from contact with bisexual partners, or having once been homosexual and being infected; or being careless in their health and sexual activities and the ones they have sex with!! While poor diet can play a role in several ways I believe the main root is a spiritual and emotional one. Spiritually, one is not connected enough with the Reality of God to be in touch with True Morality - there are things in life you can and cannot do!!! If one has not been in Touch with God, one cannot be in touch with their "True Self!" If they were, they would Feel the Signs of Right and Wrong Behavior and See these in Others!! Emotionally - feelings of self-worth (made harder with lack of good diet and habits) and results of dealings with the opposite sex, could lead one to go astray (to the other side) ... it always comes back to us, how we lead our lives, and treat each other.

There are many strong healing foods and processes along with current medication in lessening doses, and a return to a more normal sexuality, could probably lead to a breakthrough in the Cure of AIDS!!!

E.   <u>Alcohol and Drugs</u> (illegal and legal) Misuse - if our diet did its job, we would not have these problems. How many times after eating lunch do you feel like sleeping when you have important tasks at hand? Ideally after eating any meal one should take a break and rest, a short walk, then to the task at hand.

But in these torqued out times that is not considered and may be scoffed at! So, most have turned into chemists, creating their common day "Elixirs and Potions" to "get themselves right" in order to maintain and keep moving on! Very few though have the Control and Intelligence to keep it just right and the few that do miscalculate the side effects of many ingredients the body was not designed to ingest. They will work for a while, but will succumb to the "Law of Diminishing Returns" ... it always does! The dilemma is that the less serious people can see no other ways than pretty much what they are doing, except maybe tighten it up a bit more. Every action though has an equal and opposite reaction. For example the alcohol used for "a pick-me up" after a heavy meal or at the end of the work day will do that, though somewhat erratically, but the next day you reap the hangover, a little more damage to the body, and a need to soothe the stomach with heavy & greasy foods. For alcohol partakers this is a repetitive cycle: after heavy meal to up the energy, take alcohol, which temporarily stimulates the circulation and gives a psychological boost. The next day, or later on, coat the inner rawness with heavy & greasy foods.

To put it more bluntly - the alcohol, like a solvent, cuts the grease, boosts the energy and psyche; then to soothe the damage done eat heavy or greasy food & Deal w/ the Mental Aspects of the Hangover! The 'Alcoholics Anonymous' could learn something very important here, about some of the real causes of alcoholism and how the physical affects the mental. Also, the old adage "once an alcoholic, always an alcoholic" could evolve with a better understanding of the above and **that until you can control something you will never overcome it, is better than blindly abstaining from something with fear!!** "Alcoholics" need to wean themselves from their drink while improving their diet!

Make healthy drinks also, like blend some fresh grapes and a little ginger root with your wine (a good combination as you know where wine comes from – the grapes) and with straight alcohol blend fresh fruit or veggies but never together - most know how to make these drinks but not why ... be creative and you will still get your buzz, just a healthier one, until you do not need it anymore, or as much! The same holds true with illegal drug users, abusers - get a better understanding of proper diet and how an improper diet was a major cause of their problem and at the same time wean themselves from their habit. This point though there's a major stumbling block in understanding - the natural plant sources that their drugs are made from are seen as the culprit and are eradicated by drug enforcement forces! Specifically, coca plants (cocaine), poppy plants (heroin), and marijuana (smoking marijuana) were put here by God as medicinal plants with the right way to use them! The wrong way is to highly refine them and to smoke, snort, or inject them ... then you have the problems that follow!! I am not all that familiar with legal drug use, as in prescribed pharmaceuticals.

As we are talking in this segment with misuse, I would say the problem stems from not following doctor orders, or once you see how the drug(s) work, use them as a continual crunch, instead of a temporary medication until you become well!! To become well takes more than medicine, one needs a Greater Understanding of the Whole Problem that created their illness. Then go about the various ways of real, Total Healing!! All three of these areas - alcohol, illegal drug and legal drug misuse, while affecting the abusers, can also be a major root of crime and other disturbances, which affect all of society!! For a good time now the Laws of the Land have focused on alcohol and drug abuse, but these are offshoots of a greater problem - an Improper Diet & Subsequent Habits!! Can the mainstream handle this truth??!! As I have said before it all boils down to energy - how do you feel ... **the MainstreamDiet is not doing its job!!!**

F.   Mental, Emotional, and Spiritual Illness - (all interrelate with each other as well as the physical. I will be brief and to the point because books could be (and have been) written about each of these and my point in this chapter is to show a general relationship between diseases). Mental - I have seen many elderly mentally ill people, especially in nursing homes, with large lower abdomens pulling their whole body down. Clogged and constipation, how could the mind ever receive its nourishment and energy? I remember one elderly lady remarking, when asked if she needed anything, that she needed a "good movement" - as in bowel! This happens over a lifetime and some problems we have as children we never grow out of of. A young sluggish or hyper mind could lead to many mental problems: learning and understanding disabilities, disorientation, worry and self-doubt, nervousness and hyperactivity, to name a few.

During the course of one's life if not correctly solved, these could intensify especially with some pharmaceuticals, with other side effects, and one's self-prescribed solutions! Mental illness can occur at any age and in many forms, some of which may catch some by surprise ... like always trying to control others so you will feel safe or better than them; by not being open enough to share a general friendship or camaraderie with your fellow Souls, Earthlings, and Neighbors, even if you do not know them! We are all in this together and we all need to make it, for everyone is just as important to themselves as you are to yourself!!! Emotional - as children most express how they feel immediately, and a lot of times too much, perhaps because they are uncomfortable with how they feel due to hypertension from unbalanced sugar laden foods and beverages; stuffiness from clogged lungs and sinuses; and full stomach from too many heavy foods and slow moving bowels.

Expressing and feeling our different emotions is most healthy when done in a proper way, so as not to hurt or bother someone else. Whereas repressing and not feeling our emotions is unhealthy and can lead to outbursts or introversions, which can intensify and mutate, if left unresolved, as we grow older. Generally speaking, you do not really live if you do not feel and share! Emotions tie in directly with the lungs and heart and they can adversely affect each other - repressed emotions can constrict the breathing or clogged breathing can inhibit the emotions. On the other hand, a good cry or laugh can ease the heart, chest and mind!!! Spiritual - life in these times is much too difficult to go it alone, without God. Without God, we carry too much burden to understand and can become Sick with Despair! Without God you have no base for True Spiritual Understanding; without spiritual understanding how can you love and have compassion day in and out?

I once had a conversation with a Baptist Preacher, about how I felt that the idea of the Separation between Church and State was absurd. How can you govern without the church (our best ideas about God and Life)? I added that the government controlled the people more than the

Church's Influence and had Power over the Church! His last remark to me was that, God is in Control!! Thank you Pastor Leroy Brown of Trinity, Texas, that understanding has comforted me many times!! The only thing though is life is a very serious learning experience and God pretty much, lets us "Reap what we Sow" regardless of the outcome!! A very good way to learn, but must we learn the Final Lessons of Love and Harmony through Hardship and Sorrow...it's the way we're headed!!!

I feel the "Mass Consciousness" also is a constant Prayer to God, as the Energy of God is Omnipresent throughout Creation! Hence, one reason for many of our natural disasters - earthquakes, hurricanes, tornadoes, droughts, floods, pestilence, etc.

Reaping what the Mass Consciousness Sows!! Other reasons being our polluting habits, underground nuclear testing, and depleting earth's natural lubrication of oil! Now weathermen and geologists may disagree, but with so many answers eluding us, Think Deeply and Pray about These Ideas ... The Earth used to be Flat, you know!!! Worry and Stress, and the resulting offshoots from the above, is a Spiritual Illness that can reach epidemic proportions at times. So, for those who do not believe, look at the Sky and Earth around you, and then see what you can create?! It is all here for us and set in motion - the way the universe works and the way our bodies work. Take heed, be thankful, slow down, and Seek New and Higher Realities!

For we are still All God's Family, whether you believe it or not, and most likely if you do not believe, you may be adding to a serious situation that is at hand!!!

With a note of hope, I will end this chapter. I believe I have discovered some specific foods that would directly nourish certain areas of the body, including the different organs. These would be instrumental, along with the best ideas in modern conventional medicine, in treating those with heart problems or cancers in any area, as well as any other disease or illness! That is another book though and most of all some cooperative research with the Mainstream Powers that be!!! The "Fire of Hope" needs to be lit in many areas, for all people, then we can really rise up!

Yes, I feel there still is time to Bring this Earth back Home!! The Changes must Come, without delay, Dear People how We've got to Pray!!

CHAPTER 11

My Vision for our Future

If there ever was a time when one could say ' These are the Days'...
well ,'These are the Days' !! I don't believe ever before in history that
the world has been in such chaos! We seem to take for granted all of
the technology and ease of life innovations that helps to make our lives
comfortable and exciting, yet we can't seem to co-exist with each other
for very long in a relative peace!! In the last several years there have
been very severe earthquakes, volcanoes, floods, forest fires,
tornadoes, hurricanes, droughts, and a new phenomena called a
tsunami!! Most think that these are natural occurrences and not related
at all to the human condition; in other words that "We do Reap what
the Mass Consciousness Sows"! Like it or not, we live in a Self
Correcting World, or Universe, and at some point We All Must
Assume this Personal Responsibility if things are ever to get better!
Add to this mass consciousness, our terrible pollution problems
(although great strides are being and have been made, a lot of damage
has been and is being done still); and throw in a few dozen
underground nuclear bomb tests of the past (I wonder what affect
those might have with earthquakes and volcanoes as they are
awesomely powerful and generate a tremendous heat, not to mention
dangerous radiations), and we've exasperated our earthly
predicament!! Has there ever been so many wars as in the past few
decades... Iraq and Afghanistan, as always the Middle East, Somalia,
Iran, Bosnia, Hutu's and Tutsi's, and many more?! What makes These
Days more different than the Atrocities of the Past, is simply the
Extreme Power of the Myriad of Weapons Systems around Our Earth,
along w/ most of the World in a Max Stress Out!!!

One of our problems is we are way too busy and occupied to see all
what is happening, along w/ the oft neglected Deeper Insight of Life &
the Realities in which we 'choose to exist' [Until Tragedy once again
Strikes & slaps us into Sanity & Humbleness]!!! In the Great Book

called Holy Bible, Revelations speaks of the time when there will be Wars and Rumors of Wars, Floods and Droughts, & Earthquakes, but do not be alarmed for the end is not yet to come… well those that have Eyes to See and Ears to Hear, this is our Wake Up Call! Do not panic, but do not waste your time, we need to better solve our problems, sooner than later!! As I've said many times, many of our problems have a root in how we Nourish and Sustain ourselves - if we don't feel good, how can we ever act right consistently - and it usually doesn't take much to set something off!! Again, there are many other reasons Beyond Diet for our problems, but it's a major one along w/ their Subsequent Habits!

If the Disharmony & Chaos of the above escalates to melt down proportions, figuratively and literally, we have what I call "the Armageddon of Darkness" and what many current day churches believe is inevitable… although they have the " Rapture Escape Clause" in which they will be taken safely way, while the unsaved (the rest of God's Family) perishes in Eternal Damnation with, as some would say, everyday being worse than the day before until their soul is no more!! I say, these Sowers of Fear and Guilt amongst the weak minded will have a price to pay when they Meet their Maker!! How many good people have been killed already in the myriad of ways that devolve on our earth? If God is going to save you, why not them? However, like my Dad once told me, The Churches also serve important functions which societies depend upon like Marriages, Funerals, Christenings, and as a Gathering Place for Prayer and Worship in ones chosen Vein of Spirituality. Also, there is a lot of Power in the Church when many are gathered there in good purpose!!

But, I hold the Churches of this Earth **Greatly Responsible** to come to a better consensus amongst each other, because they are the Teachers of Peace and Love! **It is their Innate Responsibility to rise above their Dogma and Disagreements & into a Deeper Understanding of Holiness and sway the Balance of Power out of the hands of the Government's, the Military's, and the powers of Economics!!**

The Earth is our Home and we have got a lot of messes to clean up - we could really make this Earth a Paradise once again & have what I call the **Armageddon of the Light**!! It's like the beginning of the Holiday Season when people gradually become friendlier with each other and a New / Old Spirit Resurfaces. If we could take this special time and find out how & why it works, nurture and expand it, we could solve all our problems and eventually have a better time doing it! At the Core of this Special Time is Love and Harmony, *[which must be considered and practiced in order to evolve it]*... **Practice does make Better!!** But, in today's beta-drive, super production, fill in all the time world, we don't give it **its valuable due**! We've become schizoid, paranoid, overly defensive, way too controlling and dysfunctional, too much of the time with each other, as Our Train Barrels down the Vortex to Oblivion!!

In conclusion I return to the <u>Diet and Arthritis Cure</u>: the Carnivorous Diet will never give you Peace for very long, there will always be something gnawing at you or an anxiety that I've noticed amongst the meat eaters - they're never had ease for very long~ One reason is that the **shock of the slaughtered animal** is forever locked into its meat; and meat and animal byproducts were never meant / ordained for consumption... so Malfunctions in different ways will Occur!!

As far as the Arthritis Cure goes, if I'm given a chance to prove it and show that it will work, it could **help** set off a New Healing Revolution ... finally a 'Cure for Something' that has plagued humankind for eons! The Hope that this could create could be incredible, and with Hope comes Excitement, and with Excitement the Energy to harmoniously start finding the solutions for our many other problems: other diseases; new and cheaper and nonpolluting energy sources; poverty, crime, wars, etc..; God the Money, Time, and Worry we put toward these Problems... " **"Seek ye First the Kingdom of Heaven and All else will be Given"**, works every time!! I don't see a lot of hope in the many faces that I see and sometimes turn from daily, so obviously many things that are in place are not working! So, it's time to give New, Fresh Ideas a Chance and help create the **"Armageddon of the Light"**... *then and only then,* will the **2nd Coming** our **True Christ Selves**, have a chance to begin... The **3rd Millennium** has already begun, the **Thousand Years of Peace** prophesied, *is not off to a good start...* **As a Man / Woman Thinketh - So It Will Be...** **AMEN**

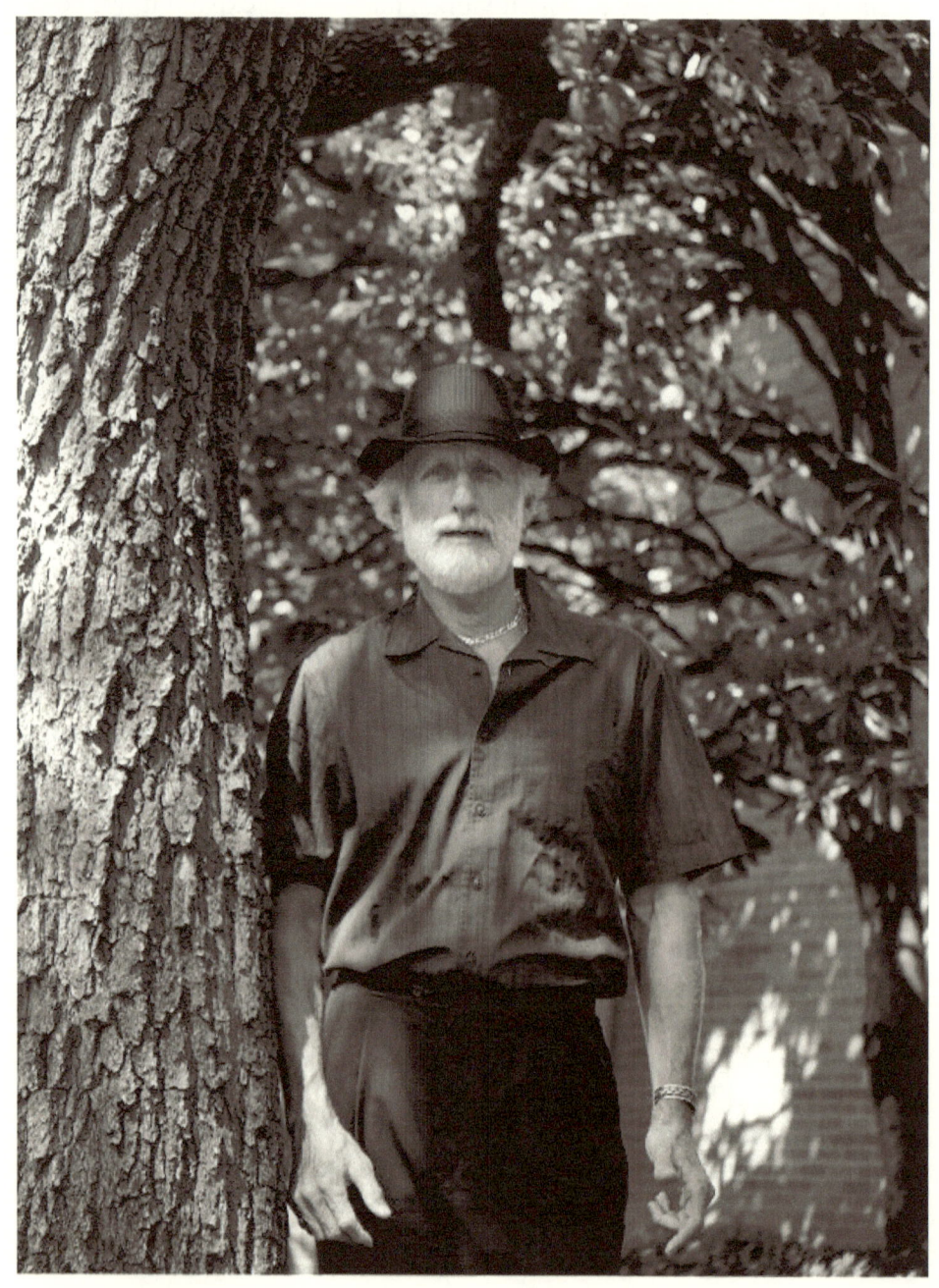

Michael Burge -- <mbrgaw2000@yahoo.com>